"As someone who continues to deal with anxiety, I found *The Fix Your Anxiety Handbook* to be most helpful. 'Anxiety is not who you are, but what you have.' This clarification, and the advice which follows, has given me some very useful tools to acknowledge and separate those anxious feelings when the monster rears its ugly head from the reality of a situation. This book is a valuable tool in the ongoing struggle to stay the course of healthy mental emotions. Stay strong, brothers and sisters!"

—ADAM FERRARA, ACTOR / COMEDIAN

"Faust Ruggiero has it right! The demon or dragon that keeps so many people from attaining their life goals must be slayed and incapacitated. Faust Ruggiero lays out the perfect plan for destroying this beast. This is a wonderful handbook for anybody who wants to move ahead in life."

—DANIEL ROEBUCK, ACTOR

"Faust was a guest on my podcast and everyone loved his concepts on improving life. His book is practical, and would help any person struggling. Thank you, Faust, for the work you do!"

—ELISA JORDANA, RADIO PERSONALITY, MUSICIAN,
COMEDY WRITER

"Anxiety can hold us back in what we want to do in life, and Faust Ruggiero's handbook on anxiety is a fantastic tool to overcome those times and help you take back control!"

—TAYLOR DAYNE, SINGER, SONG WRITER

"Faust Ruggiero possesses an abundance of information, and has created program to treat depression that I have never seen before. He has insights into the dynamics of depression, and communicates them in a way that anyone can understand and apply."

—GEORGE NOORY, COAST TO COAST RADIO HOST

THE FIX YOUR ADDICTION HANDBOOK

Bringing you out of a life of weakness and dependence and into a world of freedom and sanity

FAUST RUGGIERO, M.S.

FYHB PUBLISHING

Disclaimer: This book is designed to help you understand the dynamics of anger and provide helpful steps to assist you in your attempts to reduce its impact on your life. Before attempting to incorporate the information and action steps in this book, consult a physician to be sure that you are physically, emotionally, and intellectually capable of including the program in your life.

Published by:
FYHB Publishing
BANGOR, PA
www.faustruggiero.com

ISBNs:
Paperback: 978-1-7343830-8-9
Ebook: 978-1-7343830-9-6

Cover and interior design by Gary A. Rosenberg
www.thebookcouple.com

Printed in the United States of America

Contents

The Practical Road Map to Sobriety:
An Opportunity to Fix Your Life

Introduction

DO YOU WANT TO UNDERSTAND THE VARIOUS TYPES of addiction, reduce addiction's impact on your life, and eventually free yourself from its paralyzing effects? If so, *The Fix Your Addiction Handbook* is for you. This is book five in The Fix Yourself Empowerment Series. It follows the award-winning *The Fix Yourself Handbook*, which debuted in December 2019; the much-heralded *The Fix Your Anxiety Handbook*, published in June 2023; *The Fix Your Depression Handbook*, published in December 2023; and *The Fix Your Anger Handbook*, published in December 2024.

Consistent with the approach taken in the first four volumes in the series, the program is presented as a process journey. All the books in The Fix Yourself Empowerment Series are written as journeys. I do this because I want you to understand that life is a journey, and by going slow and understanding the processes associated with it, you can learn how to live a happy and productive life. Also, by presenting the program as a life journey, I can give you a glimpse of what your life can be like during the latter stages of the journey—that is, what your life can look like if you stay committed to what you read here.

I present the information about addiction this way to help you understand what is happening to your body, your mind, and your emotions. I want you to be able to separate yourself from this harrowing way of living life. I also want you to get a clearer picture of what has happened to you throughout your life as your world-shattering addiction started becoming a dominant force in your life. When addiction takes hold of your life, it overwhelms you, making it difficult for you to understand what is happening to you. It is important to understand the dynamics of addiction, what type of addiction you have, how it manifests, and what you can do to reduce its impact on your life.

Each bite-size chapter presents the necessary information you need to understand a specific dynamic about the condition. The route addiction follows as it overtakes your life is discussed, and the precise steps to help you correct the problem are provided as the chapters wind down. I have designed this program so you may apply the steps to your circumstances as they exist in your life. However, as you will see, the problems presented here can be experienced by anyone who suffers from addiction or whose life has been affected by someone who is addicted. You are not as different as you think, and there is a logical way out of your distress.

Consistent with all the books in The Fix Yourself Empowerment Series, *The Fix Your Addiction Handbook* is the product of more than thirty years of practical counseling application. Being certified in addiction treatment, I have been working with addicts for over forty years. I developed the program, researched it extensively, and successfully used it with my clients. It is a dynamic addition to an existing counseling program, or if you have difficulty obtaining professional counseling, it can provide you with either a viable alternative or an introduction to that step.

Each chapter in The Fix Yourself Empowerment Series opens with a quote that offers a glimpse into the chapter's content. This is followed by the specific processes to employ (see page 10), which will help you do the work to alleviate the problem addressed in the chapter. I have included the processes to be used as program supports to help you work with all the information and suggestions I am making. The processes are tools you can use to implement each program step. As you proceed through the program and secure the assistance of a counselor and support people to help you reduce addiction's impact on your life, these processes can be included in your discussions with them, and they will help you make the changes discussed in this book. A few processes— Brutal Honesty, I Over E, Present-Understand-Fix, and Slowing Down Life's Pace—appear in each chapter because they are foundational to the entire program.

There are fifty-two processes in the Process Way of Life program. However, not all of them will directly apply to addiction. The initial fifty-two processes were included in each chapter of *The Fix Yourself Handbook*, the program's flagship book. In that book, the text was written to address many different problems on the human spectrum. All fifty-two processes were needed to navigate the program presented in the book. In the subsequent books, only the processes that directly apply to the information discussed in the chapter will be used. So don't be concerned if not all the processes are used in this book.

I have kept the chapters short and to the point with direct and concise information. I have found this is the best way to ensure the information is understood, especially when addiction can have such a dramatic impact on your life and the lives of those close to you. Since the book can be used as a reference guide should you need it in the future, the design makes it easier to refer back to each chapter if you need to refresh yourself at a later date.

As each chapter concludes, you will find the "Time to Take Action" sections. Here, I present the steps I advise you to take to help alleviate the problem examined in that chapter. I always provide action steps in everything I teach because information without a workable course of action can rarely be applied. These action steps are the fuel that makes the program run. I have also provided you with a declaration at the end of each chapter. These affirmations will help you maintain your enthusiasm as you continue addressing the issues in the chapter. The chapter closes with a short introduction of what will be covered in the next chapter.

As you move forward in your life, it will be important for you to embrace the concept of information-gathering and fact-finding. Correct information always leads to the potential for a solution. With this in mind, Chapters 1 and 2 provide the important general information you need to understand about addiction. Chapters 3 through 18 are designed to explain the different types of addiction. It is vital to read these chapters carefully because they will provide you with the foundational information you need to create an efficient plan to address your addiction. The progression of the addiction (from user to addict), its hold on the addict, and the collateral damage are discussed in each chapter.

Chapters 19 through 29 begin building your treatment plan to reduce addiction's impact on your life. These chapters provide you with specific features of a workable plan to help you reduce and, if possible, recover from the addiction that has plagued your life and those close to you, as well as the steps you need to take to formulate that plan and begin your process of recovery from this horrifying nemesis.

Chapter 28 provides the information you need to live in the new world you are creating. Many people do their best to end their pain and move into a new way of life, but it can be challenging to stay there since it is unfamiliar ground, and they do not have an efficient plan to live there. This chapter provides you with the information to do just that. Chapter 29 provides a viable plan to help you maintain the gains you have made in your recovery from addiction.

The book provides the initial tools to help you move beyond your addiction. It will always be available as a reference guide and a lifelong support ally. Consistent with any program I design and implement, it is not meant to be a quick-fix problem-solver. This is a lifelong program designed to provide the information you need to help you move beyond your addiction and live a happy and healthy life.

For those of you who have read the first four installments of The Fix Yourself Empowerment Series, you may note that I am advising considerably more involvement with professional counselors and support people in this book. Addiction demands a daily step-by-step program, which is the key component of the recovery process. You will need people like program guides, counselors, and other addiction professionals to help you begin your recovery program and maintain the gains you are making.

If you are willing to give this program your time and commitment, it will become an invaluable part of your everyday life. You are greater than the addiction that has been defining your life. You are great! So get ready to become the master of your destiny. Prepare yourself for a life-changing program. There is a way out of your addiction—and this is that way! Follow me.

HOW TO READ THIS BOOK

The Fix Your Addiction Handbook and the program that supports it is a program for life, and nothing about it should ever move quickly. I advise that you read each chapter slowly. Think about what you have read and how you can apply the information in the chapter, especially if the type of addiction covered in Chapters 3 through 18 pertains to your current circumstances. Move to the next chapter when you think you understand what you have read. Regardless of what type of addiction has entered your life, you can find information about it in Chapters 3 through 18. Chapters 19 through 29 present the program any addict, family member, and, for that matter, anyone interested in increasing the quality of their life can use.

I have presented most of the information in the book in general terms so that it may be understood by addicts and those close to them who are trying to understand the addiction. At times, however, I will speak directly to the addict and/or to family members. This will help you understand the information more efficiently and apply it to yourselves and/or your family members and significant others when necessary.

Some people find reading each chapter two or three times important. Doing so can help them better understand the information provided. Sharing what you read with family and close friends is a good idea. If you already have a counselor, a 12-step sponsor, or other support people, share it with them.

Addiction can be a difficult condition to beat, but it is not impossible to do so. Take your time with the program and apply the action steps in your life. Let others be there to counsel and support you as you take the steps to rid yourself of the addiction that has controlled you so that you may live the happy life that has been waiting for you. Since addiction can have such a profound effect on your ability to understand what you are reading, it's a good idea to share this book with a close friend who can help you understand and interpret the information I am presenting.

NOTE: The sole purpose of the information in this book is to help you understand the dynamics of addiction and suggest some healthy alternatives to help you begin a program that can assist you in restoring sanity to your world. Before starting any program, consult your physician to determine if there is any reason to avoid it or if changes in your medical program need to be made before you start.

THE PROCESSES—CATEGORIES AND DESCRIPTIONS

	Process	Description
1	**Personal Inventory** (Alternate and/or related terms: *Internal Focus, Morality*)	The process of focusing our energy inward to allow for the identification of personal strengths and self-understanding, with the goal of understanding our personal principles concerning the distinction between right and wrong.
2	**Slow and Steady** (Alternate and/or related terms: Patience, Slowing Down Life's Pace, Incremental Forward Movement)	The movement away from quick and impulsive behaviors, and into a state of willful tolerance of delay through the deceleration of a lifestyle that leads to poor decisions and internal conflict, with the understanding that only through small, well-planned steps can we create sustained change and improve the quality of our lives.
3	**Honesty** (Alternate and/or related terms: *Brutal Honesty, Humility, Truth-Telling*)	The process of being absolutely honest with ourselves, even to the point of personal discomfort, and choosing to take a modest view of our own importance for the purposes of opening oneself up to personal growth.
4	**I Over E** (Intellect over Emotion) (Alternate and/or related terms: *Emotional Control, Fact-Finding, Intelligent Decision-Making*)	Taking the steps necessary to reduce the impact of emotions on our intellectual processes and using our intellect to exhaustively search for the facts in situations that may lead to stress and personal problems, before our emotions have an opportunity to distort them. Cultivating the understanding that knowledge must be applied so it may become a parameter of personal growth.
5	**Present-Understand-Fix** (Alternate and/or related terms: *Fact-Finding*)	The formula we will use in every chapter to address your problems. We present the problem, we use the facts to understand it, and we take the steps to fix it.

6	**Surrendering to the Process** (Alternate and/or related terms: Trust, Faith, Belief, Honor, Dignity)	The willingness to have unconditional trust, either in a process or some unknown entity, such as a higher power, and to allow ourselves to become subservient to the processes, so that we can learn to believe in ourselves, knowing we are capable of being the person we want to be. Having learned to do this, we can learn to think, feel, and behave in a fashion that raises our consciousness to higher-order thoughts and feelings and connects us to our innermost spirit.
7	**Effective Communication** (Alternate and/ or related terms: Warm Confrontation, Positive Language Reciprocity, Communication, Conflict Resolution, Listening)	Understanding and mastering the art of positive information exchanges. The ability to gather the facts, understand them, place them in an internally cohesive framework and present that framework, intelligently, to others to address problems. Learning to listen to ourselves, and to others, even if the information presents challenges. Understanding that the way we speak to ourselves and to others can set the stage for how we feel about ourselves and how we communicate with others.
8	**Cleaning House** (Alternate and/or related terms: Life Inventory, Eliminating Toxic People, Housekeeping, Gatekeeping, Boundary-Setting)	The honest review of one's life and those relationships in it. The removal of all people, events, and situations that may cause pain, conflict, confusion, or dysfunction from one's life to make way for positive and functional information and life-enhancing processes, followed by the practice of monitoring who and what may enter our lives thereafter. Setting boundaries regarding who gets in and how close, and learning to defend those boundaries.

9	**Simplifying Life** (Alternate and/or related terms: Life on Life's Terms, Keeping Life Simple, Life's Natural Flow)	Understanding how to apply life's natural flow in our lives, along with the removal of any irrational, unreasonable expectations, and unnecessary complexity from life to make room for a simpler and more productive way of living.
10	**Living the Journey** (Alternate and/ or related terms: Reduction of Destination Living, One-Day-at-a-Time Living, Living in the Moment, Journey Living, Creativity, Passion, Humor)	Releasing one's attachment to a happiness in life that is dependent on one's arrival at specific, magnificent destinations in favor of focusing on the present, with minimum movement back to past people and events, or forward to events which have not yet occurred. The willingness to focus all life energy on our present life and happiness, moment by moment, as life is being lived, and to appreciate the lighter sides of life, thus reducing stress and pain.
11	**Closure on the Past** (Alternate and/ or related terms: *Settling Past Issues, Forgiveness*)	Judiciously reviewing all past situations and events to put closure on them. Once we've done this, we undertake a step-by-step process to understand what we and others have done wrong, to make amends, and allow ourselves to move forward with reduced emotional pain; forgiving ourselves and others who may have hurt us.
12	**Eyes on the Prize** (Alternate and/ or related terms: *Goal-Setting, Time/ Energy Management, Learning to Be Comfortable with Being Uncomfortable, Risk-Taking*)	The practice of setting a long-term goal, complete with short-term goals, action steps, and an executable plan to carry them out in a coherent, cohesive, and timely fashion, and then consciously managing our daily clock and applying our energy to healthy modes of thought and behavior. Change, by definition, is unsettling. Temporary, uncomfortable time frames lead to the happiness and fulfillment we seek. That is where understanding and growth live.

13	**Commitment** (Alternate and/or related terms: *Journey Living, Trust, Faith*)	Enduring dedication. The Process Way of Life takes time, and continuous, unwavering commitment to the program is essential to ensure its success.
14	**Service** (Alternate and/or related terms: *Being in Service*)	The willingness to turn our rewards outward to help serve the needs of others without expectation of notoriety or payback.
15	**Wisdom** (Alternate and/or related terms: *Sustained Learning, Humility*)	Being committed to remaining an eternal student of life's lessons and positive teaching sources so we can reach our goal of having the experience, knowledge, and good judgment to achieve an understanding of the bigger picture in life and how to apply ourselves there.
16	**Gratitude** (Alternate and/or related terms: *Trust, Faith, Belief, Honor, Dignity*)	The understanding that we must be grateful for all we are, all we have, and all we can be, and that we must express this in every moment of our lives.
17	**Maintaining the Program** (Alternate and/or related terms: *System Maintenance, Housekeeping*)	The establishment and maintenance of an internally balanced power source where the intellect, emotions, body, and spirit become one. This power source is always alive and functional, emanating from inside ourselves.
18	**Internal Balance**	This is the goal of the program. It is the point where our physical, intellectual, emotional, and spiritual attributes operate in a state of enhanced equilibrium.
19	**Pure Love**	That point in the Process Way of Life where, through internal balance, we allow our new power source to be realized, to wrap itself around all we feel, touch, see, and do. This is love at its purest level.

◇◇◇◇◇◇◇◇◇◇◇◇

CHAPTER 1

Addiction—A Simple Introductory Primer

It is the surrender of the body and the will as it takes ownership of your life and your world.

PROCESSES TO EMPLOY: Brutal Honesty, I Over E, Present-Understand-Fix Slowing Down Life's Pace, Internal Focus, Fact-Finding

---

THERE ARE MANY FORMS OF ADDICTION. Some people are addicted to alcohol and other drugs; others fall prey to gambling, sex, or food addiction. "Addiction," as I am defining it, is *a chronic, relapsing disorder characterized by obsessive thinking and compulsive behaviors with little regard for the potential adverse consequences.* Medical science considers addiction a brain disorder because it involves functional changes to brain circuits involved in reward, stress, and control. Satisfying the addiction provides immediate gratification, though the physical and neurological changes may last long after a person has entered into recovery.

Addiction is not unlike other diseases, such as cancer or heart disease. It can disrupt the normal, healthy functioning of all the body's systems and organs and seriously harm a person's mind and emotions. If left untreated, it can last a lifetime and may lead to unrelenting pain and suffering and, for some, premature death. One cannot discount the powerful influence addiction has over the body. Consequently, addiction diagnosis and treatment must take into account the physical aspects of the problem. *In treating addiction, it is important to treat the whole person.* This will become apparent as we proceed.

HAND-ME-DOWNS

For decades, research has indicated a genetic predisposition to addiction. These studies have primarily focused on alcohol and other drugs. I define "genetic predisposition" as the *increased likelihood of developing a particular physical/neurological condition based on the presence of one or more genetic variants and/or a family history.* Today, we are more knowledgeable about the way addiction works. Instead of simply focusing on addictions related to substance abuse, the focus is on a more global approach to genetic predisposition. This means that being predisposed can apply to a broader variety of addictions, as you will discover.

An example of a predisposition to an addiction might be someone who comes from an alcoholic background, where at least one biological parent was an alcoholic. The likelihood of their children being predisposed to alcohol increases when one parent carries that genetic variant. It increases significantly if both parents carry the variant. Another example might be a parent who is a workaholic. Their children could also be workaholics because the genetic predisposition comes from the genetic variant predisposing the brain to demonstrate compulsive behaviors that can find their way into the work environment.

Predisposition does not necessarily mean that a child will have the same "drug of choice" as their parents. By "drug of choice," I am referring to the object of obsessive-compulsive behaviors. This means that one or both parents may be substance abusers, but their children may become addicted to another substance or another activity. So, a person who is an alcoholic may have children who are also predisposed to addiction, but the focus of their addiction is some other substance, object, or behavior. The behavior could be gambling or sex, or it might find its way into another substance like prescription or street drugs.

There are times when I have treated people who are addicted, but I can find no family history of addiction. So, genetic anomalies coming from parents do not always mean that they will transfer to the children, Although, more often than not, a family history of addiction does increase the likelihood of some addiction in future generations.

Treatment plans should always be formulated with an understanding of one's family history, assuming that it is available. As research has progressed, it has generated the use of genetic testing that can provide valuable insights into the correlation between one's family history and the possibility of addiction being a part of one's life. Also, the type of addiction that one's parents had can have some relevance regarding specific elements in the treatment plan.

Another important factor is the person's mental health. Once again, there are genetic markers that can predispose someone to mental health conditions. Conditions like depression, anxiety, attention deficit disorder (ADD), and bipolar disorder can increase the possibility of involvement in addictive thoughts and behaviors that can lead to or exacerbate existing addictions. There is also a circular relationship between mental health and addiction. Sometimes, one's mental health causes involvement in addictive behaviors or makes them worse. At other times, it is the addiction that instigates mental health issues.

ENVIRONMENTALLY SPEAKING

Genetics can play a significant role in whether someone is predisposed to addiction. However, one's environment can also impact the onset of addiction and how severe it can become. The Harvard Twin Study of Substance Abuse demonstrated the correlation between genetic coding and the environment on the potential for substance abuse. The study stated, "Our research has demonstrated significant influences by genetic, shared environmental, and unique environmental factors on the abuse of illicit substances. Multivariate analyses have indicated that the co-occurrence of abuse of various types of illicit drugs reflects a common vulnerability, influenced by both genetic and environmental factors, that cuts across all categories of illicit drugs.[1]

Though someone can be genetically predisposed to become addicted, this does not necessarily mean that they will become an addict. There are many instances of one or more parents who are addicted but have children who are not. Likewise, some parents are not addicted, but they may have one or more children who are. In these cases, the addict's environment, more than their genetics, likely led to their addiction issues.

When a person has a genetic predisposition and their environment supports the addictive cycle, the chances of them becoming addicted significantly increase. More often than not, when a person displays addictive tendencies, there are both genetic and environmental markers involved in the development of the addiction. Usually, a genetically predisposed person will have a propensity to become addicted, and their environment becomes a supportive device, one that enables and nurtures the addiction. The role of nature and nurture—that is, how genetics and or the environment may influence addiction—is precisely the reason why family and medical histories are so essential in the diagnosis and treatment of addiction. The more information we have about a person's familial and medical history and environmental influences, the more efficient the treatment plan can be.

BRAIN IN THE GAME

In each book in the Fix Yourself Empowerment Series, I have discussed how powerful the human brain is, how it works to keep you happy, and how conniving it can be. As you will see as we proceed, the addicted brain becomes highly skilled in the art of manipulation when addiction becomes part of your life. Whether or not you are predisposed to addiction, when your brain experiences the euphoria, control, diversionary behaviors, and other quasi-benefits an addiction offers, it will tenaciously guard that addiction and help you keep it active.

The human brain does everything it can to keep us in an eudaemonic state while at the same time doing its best to avoid its infelicific counterpart. "Eudaemonic" is defined as "producing happiness," and infelicific" is defined as "producing unhappiness." The addicted mind is in a continuous state of pleasure-seeking and does its best to avoid any form of conflict or discomfort. It lives according to the pleasure principle and will do its best to give its owner as much euphoria as possible.

Addicts can become master manipulators. Think of addiction as though it is a full-time job and that you are obsessed with every aspect of the work. This is the way the human mind processes addiction. The addiction is always in control, and the strategies of the mind are both to keep it active and to hide it from the rest of the world. It maximizes its defenses, goes on the offense when necessary, and has a single-minded approach to keep you euphoric and distracted as it does its best to put distance between you and the discomfort that comes from withdrawal when the drug or behavior is not accessible.

As magnificent as the brain is, it doesn't take long for an addiction to overpower its sense of reasoning and healthy living. When dependence on the drug or behavior develops, your brain can quickly lose focus on your physical, emotional, intellectual, and spiritual health. The majority of its resources are now being applied to maintaining the heightened state of euphoria along with the significantly reduced pain response that the addiction provides. Now, at all costs, and often without consideration of the damage to yourself or others, the addiction takes control of your brain and, subsequently, your life.

Chapters 3 through 18 will give you an in-depth analysis of the various types of addiction. You will notice that each addiction has its specific features but that they all have the same kind of effect on your brain. In each case, your neurology changes, your body adjusts to both the euphoric state and the "rush" the addiction provides, and you are compelled to repeat the behaviors. The following gives you an idea of the addictions covered in this book. There is a chapter dedicated to each addiction and its unique challenges.

Alcohol

Alcohol is the most commonly abused substance. Socially, it is used to celebrate and to enjoy time with friends. People use it to relax at the end of a hard day, to help reduce emotional overreactions, and/or to shut off an overactive brain. Some people will have a drink or two at the end of the day, while others may drink only on weekends. For some, it becomes an obsession that develops into an addictive way of living.

Nicotine

Like alcohol, nicotine is a very commonly abused drug. Its euphoric effects are minimal and not as pronounced as with other drugs. It is one of the most addictive substances, and many people smoke for long periods before they quit. Relapses can occur often, and the behavior is often tied to daily living rituals such as after-dinner cigarettes, alcohol consumption, and smoking with a cup of coffee. While cigarette use seems to have gone down over the last five years, vaping has increased, and, along with it, the use of nicotine.

Prescription Drugs

SAMSHA reports that the use of prescription drugs has dramatically increased over the past twenty years. Drugs are prescribed for conditions like heart disease, diabetes, cancer, high blood pressure, and cholesterol reduction, to mention just a few. Also, there are those medications used for pain and anxiety. Though these medications are closely scrutinized, they are also the most often abused medications. According to The National Centers for Drug Abuse Statistics, prescription drug abuse is insidious and widely misunderstood. Young adults are the heaviest users, but older and elderly patients are at heightened risk of misuse and addiction.

Cocaine

Cocaine is a tropane alkaloid that acts as a central nervous system stimulant. It is primarily used recreationally for its euphoric and rewarding effects. Tropane alkaloids can cause blurred vision, dry mouth, drowsiness, and delirium. People who use cocaine tend to like it because, in addition to its stimulant properties, it is also a powerful euphoric. It is highly addictive and puts a tremendous strain on the nervous system and the cardiovascular system.

Amphetamines

Amphetamines are stimulant drugs. They increase the communication speed between the brain and the body. This makes the user more alert and physically active, stay awake, or perhaps study more efficiently. Athletes use them to boost their performance in sports. They are highly addictive and cause significant damage to the brain and throughout the body.

Hallucinogens

Hallucinogens are a large and diverse class of psychoactive drugs that can produce altered states of consciousness characterized by significant alterations in thought, mood, and perception. Most hallucinogens can be categorized as either psychedelics (a type of drug that changes a person's perception of reality), dissociatives (psychedelic drugs that cause detachment and hallucinations), or deliriants (drugs that cause a state of delirium). Long-term use can have a significant impact on neurological functioning.

Marijuana

Marijuana (the dried leaves, stands, and flowers of the cannabis plant produce a pleasant euphoria and a sense of relaxation in many cases. Other common effects include heightened sensory perception (e.g., seeing brighter colors), laughter, pain reduction, altered perception of time, and increased appetite. These effects can vary dramatically from person to person. The legalization of marijuana for medical and recreational purposes in many U.S. states has significantly increased its usage. Depending on the frequency of use and the potency of the product, marijuana can be addictive.

Food

Though food is not a drug, many people become addicted to detrimental eating habits. Overeating, gorging, bulimia, and anorexia are all associated with problems surrounding food. Food is often used to maintain a sense of control over one's environment and other people and to address past traumas and fears.

Gambling

It is easy to focus on winning or losing as a motivating factor in a gambling addiction. However, when I treat people with gambling addictions, they rarely talk about winning or losing. Their addiction is about the adrenaline rush that gambling produces. Where losing may stop the process since finances become depleted, winning only ensures more playing time. It is what happens during play that keeps the body, emotions, and mind engaged and produces a euphoric rush that creates the addiction.

Smartphones and Video Games

This is an addiction that so many people deny. Smartphones and other electronics create significantly higher neurological activity. The rush that they produce ranges from mild to intense, and since people rarely separate themselves from their electronics, they do not realize the power of the addiction. It is when they are separated from their device that withdrawal sets in. The withdrawal from electronics can be as powerful as any other drug. Electronics can produce the same addictive processes in the brain that we see with drug addiction.

Sex and Pornography

One of the reasons sex and pornography are so powerful is that both of them attach to primal human drives. In its most fundamental form, the human body is a sexual machine. Its physical design is to procreate and reproduce. These functions are set in the brain's pleasure center, providing euphoric pleasure that keeps a person in a state of desire, ensuring the survival of the species. However, we have evolved to the point that the need for procreation is not as pronounced as it was in more primitive times, and sex is used primarily for enjoyment. As with anything else we use for enjoyment, there can be a tendency to abuse it and to become addicted to it.

Self-Abuse

Self-abuse has many forms, and it can be painful while instigating feelings of shame, guilt, and worthlessness. Examples of self-abuse are cutting, Trichotillomania (hair pulling), and head banging, to mention just a few. Interestingly, these behaviors can develop into addiction as the brain and body adjusts to them. The addiction can be just as intense as any other; it does produce withdrawal symptoms during abstention and has a drastic effect on a person's life.

Shopping

There are far more shopaholics than most people know. Shopping addiction in its most intense form is easy to diagnose. These people are visibly committed to the process. They often have many items they have purchased but have never worn or used. Shopping is usually a diversion from pain, discomfort, or other life conditions and can replace the absence of nurturance and affection. Regardless of where it begins, it can quickly develop into an addictive process. When it does, it has all the same parameters we see in other addictions, and the withdrawal from it can be as intense as drug addiction.

Workaholism

For some, there is a separation between their work life and the rest of their lives. Others work long hours, often when they do not need to, while others routinely bring work home. Still, for others, if they are not performing duties related to their primary employment, they will either seek part-time jobs or find involved activities and projects around the house. These people often have difficulty "shutting off their brain," and staying in action keeps their minds quiet.

Exercise

Physical exercise is a very important component in maintaining a healthy body. However, when exercise ties itself to self-image, obsessive weight loss, muscle growth, etc., it can become an overindulgence in something initially designed to be productive and intellectually and emotionally fulfilling. People who are addicted to exercise will exercise for long periods, rarely, if ever, miss an exercise session, set unrealistic goals, and have body-image issues. They have difficulty understanding the need for rest as part of muscle growth and repair and are often protective and argumentative when their exercise program is challenged.

SUMMING IT UP

We have become an addiction-based society. Typically, when we look at addiction, we focus on drugs and alcohol. We primarily look at street drugs, opiates, and an overindulgence in alcohol. We are surrounded by resources and substances that can become overused. Some of those can develop into addictions and can drastically change the course of our lives. All too often, we move forward in an endeavor without thoroughly researching the information that can be so important in our decision-making process. We tend to decide what we want to do and then proceed only to discover the problems associated with that decision later.

I have always preached the notion of fact-finding before decision-making. That process is so important regarding something that can compromise the quality of your life and, in some cases, possesses the strength to end it. We have become a culture whose use of addictive substances and activities has become normalized to the point that many don't fear their consequences. Acquiring the facts about the various forms of addiction is essential to help us avoid the potential disasters they can cause.

 TIME TO TAKE ACTION

1. Do an exhaustive family background check to determine if there is a history of addiction or mental health issues in your family.

2. Obtain a medical history as it pertains to your grandparents, parents, and siblings to determine if there were/are any addiction or mental health issues.

3. Obtain all the facts you can about suicides or attempted suicides, incarcerations, hospital stays, and anything that may indicate the possibility of addiction or mental health issues in your family. If you don't know them, ask other family members if they have any information.

4. It is a good idea to make an appointment with your primary care physician. You might obtain a family history from them if they are able to provide it. A history of mental health or suicide history which is also advantageous. The more information you have, the more efficient your treatment plan can be.

 ## DRIVING IT HOME

Nothing about addiction is easy. It can be an insidious condition that begins innocently and develops into a life-threatening monster. Understanding as much as you can about genetic and environmental factors and your family history helps you acquire the information that is necessary to keep addiction from ruining your life. In the early stages, honesty is your most potent ally. Lies, defenses, misdirection, and diversions are the fuel that keeps addiction strong and prevents you from obtaining the treatment necessary to remove it from your life. This is a problem you need to face head-on. If you do so early, the chance of recovery significantly increases. Be honest with yourself, and don't let this life-shattering disease destroy your world.

YOUR DECLARATION IS: *I will become knowledgeable about addiction to keep it from destroying my life!*

 ## ONWARD

In the next chapter, I will discuss the misconceptions and realities about addiction. I will dispel the myths and present accurate information that sets the stage for what will occur as the program unfolds.

CHAPTER 2

◇◇◇◇◇◇◇◇◇◇

Myths and Realities— What Are the Facts?

There is no leeway or gray area; the facts are the facts. Knowing them can be the difference between living and dying.

PROCESSES TO EMPLOY: Brutal Honesty, I Over E, Present-Understand-Fix, Slowing Down Life's Pace, Internal Focus, Fact-Finding

---

ADDICTION IS ONE OF THOSE CONDITIONS THAT DEMANDS factual information. Without that knowledge, it can progress unaddressed long enough to cause significant damage to a person's life. Often, the warning signs for addiction are not clear, making diagnosis difficult. It is not uncommon for an addiction to progress to the point of crisis before it is identified. There are two reasons for this:

1. The person with the addiction is doing their best to hide their use and any symptoms.

2. All too often, those close to a person struggling with addiction do not have the facts that are necessary to understand what is happening.

Addiction is one of those conditions that is misunderstood, and the information about it is often incomplete or misinterpreted. The addicted person does their best to misdirect those close to them from determining the cause of their observable behavioral changes. Also, family members and close friends are usually not skilled enough and don't possess the necessary information to understand what is happening. Each type of addiction has its specific characteristics, and it is important to understand the related facts. To start your addiction education, what follows is an examination of the various types of addiction and the myths and realities associated with each.

ALCOHOL

INACCURATE—Alcohol is not a drug.

ACCURATE—Alcohol is processed by the body as a drug. That it has been legal for a significant amount of time and comes in liquid form does not negate its designation as a drug.

INACCURATE—A person has to drink every day to be considered an alcoholic.

ACCURATE—A diagnosis of alcoholism does not require daily consumption.

INACCURATE—If you only drink beer, you are probably not an alcoholic.

ACCURATE—Regardless of the drink, all alcohol is the same. It may come from different sources, and some drinks contain a higher alcohol content. You can certainly be an alcoholic even if you only drink beer.

INACCURATE—All alcoholics experience severe cravings if they are not drinking.

ACCURATE—Some alcoholics, like binge drinkers, who may only drink for a few days a week or even per month, may not experience cravings when they are not using the drug.

INACCURATE—Men are more prone to be alcoholics than women.

ACCURATE—Alcohol can progress to the point of addiction in women, the same as it does for men. More men tend to drink, and they may consume larger amounts of alcohol, but there is no research to indicate that men are more likely to be alcoholics than women.

INACCURATE—You know you are an alcoholic if you attend Alcoholics Anonymous meetings.

ACCURATE—While some alcoholics attend Alcoholics Anonymous meetings, this is the treatment for one who goes to the meetings because alcoholism is impacting their life.

INACCURATE—Alcohol is not as dangerous as other drugs.

ACCURATE—Alcohol causes damage to brain cells and has a severe impact on the liver and heart. Drinking too much in a single sitting can lead to alcohol poisoning, which can be fatal.

NICOTINE

INACCURATE—Nicotine is relatively harmless to the human body.

ACCURATE—Chronic systemic exposure to nicotine from cigarette smoking may contribute to accelerated coronary and peripheral vascular disease, acute cardiac ischemic events, delayed wound healing, reproductive disturbances, peptic ulcer disease, and esophageal reflux.

INACCURATE—Nicotine is not as addictive as street drugs.

ACCURATE—Nicotine is one of the most addictive drugs. For many people, it is the most difficult drug to quit using.

INACCURATE—Most cigarettes are made using tobacco and a few preservatives.

ACCURATE—Nicotine is a colorless, poisonous alkaloid derived from the tobacco plant. It is a powerful drug that affects the brain and quickly becomes addictive. Cigarettes often contain tar, carbon monoxide, arsenic, ammonia, acetone, toluene, methylamine, pesticides, Polonium-210, and methanol. None of these are deemed safe for human consumption.

INACCURATE—It doesn't matter whether you quit or not; the damage has already been done.

ACCURATE—When a person quits smoking, vaping, or dipping, the body immediately starts repairing itself, albeit slowly.

INACCURATE—Nicotine replacement therapy (NRT) is as harmful as smoking.

ACCURATE—NRT (patch, gum, lozenge, inhaler, and nasal spray) is much safer than using tobacco.

INACCURATE—Smoking cigarettes can relax you.

ACCURATE—All too often, the stress one feels between cigarettes is due to the withdrawal from the previous cigarette. Smoking another cigarette gives a false sense of relaxation because it addresses the withdrawal symptoms that developed after the last cigarette.

INACCURATE—Smoking "light" cigarettes does not cause the same kinds of damage as regular cigarettes.

ACCURATE—Though there may be less damage from light cigarettes, there is always damage from smoking, and over time, there isn't that much difference in the effects.

PRESCRIPTION DRUGS

INACCURATE—Prescription drugs are safe because a doctor prescribes them.

ACCURATE—All drugs have side effects. Some of them are more serious than others. Just because your physician prescribes a drug does not mean it is safe.

INACCURATE—There is nothing wrong with using someone else's prescription if you have the same problem.

ACCURATE—Everyone's body and physical conditions are different. What may be safe for one person may not necessarily be safe for someone else.

INACCURATE—Prescription drugs are safer than street drugs.

ACCURATE—Though prescription drugs are controlled and thought to be safer than street drugs, a high percentage of drug overdoses are the result of prescription drug overdoses.

INACCURATE—If you don't have the money or time to spend on doctor's visits and expensive prescriptions, ordering drugs online is a safe alternative.

ACCURATE—Ordering medications online, other than from pharmacies, is dangerous because you have no idea where those drugs came from. Also, without first consulting with a doctor, you have no idea how those medications will affect your body and their potential side effects.

INACCURATE—Opiates are the most efficient way to treat pain.

ACCURATE—It is advisable to use less drastic methods such as aspirin, acetaminophen, and ibuprofen. Though these nonprescription medications do have side effects, when used properly, they are usually not lethal. Deep tissue massage is also an efficient way to treat pain.

INACCURATE—Going "cold turkey" is the best way to cure opioid addiction.

ACCURATE—When a person is addicted to opioids and suddenly stops using or goes "cold turkey," they are likely to start experiencing opioid withdrawal symptoms. These symptoms can be severe, and trying to quit this way is associated with potentially debilitating physical consequences and a very high risk of relapse. If someone is trying to quit opioids, it is recommended that they do so with professional support to help manage symptoms and support recovery.

INACCURATE—Only people with addictions are at risk of overdosing on opioids.

ACCURATE—Anyone who abuses opioids is at risk of overdose, although some people may be at higher risk than others.

INACCURATE—Prescription drug addiction is a psychological disorder, and dependent people need better willpower.

ACCURATE—Prescription drug addiction is also a physical addiction. The body adjusts to the drug, and after a period of continued use, it can adapt and become dependent on the effects it provides. Treatment must address the physical and psychological addictions.

INACCURATE—People who become addicted to prescription drugs will always need an inpatient program to help them address their dependence on the drug.

ACCURATE—An inpatient program is not always necessary to treat prescription drug addiction. A skilled professional with an understanding of substance abuse and addiction can help with the step-down process to relieve the physical dependence on the drug. Additional counseling is advised to help with the psychological dependence. That said, at times, an inpatient program may be necessary.

HALLUCINOGENS

INACCURATE—Hallucinogens are safe recreational drugs.

ACCURATE—Consistent with the use of any drug over a significant period, long-term use of hallucinogens can cause neurological problems. They can have long-term adverse effects. There will also be an impact on organs in the body, such as the liver and kidneys, which process the drugs.

INACCURATE—Hallucinogens are great party drugs.

ACCURATE—In many cases, hallucinogenic "trips" instigate feelings of panic, anxiety, and fear, feelings that eventually subside. The nature of the trip often depends on the personality of the user, the type of drug being used, and the amount being used. Also, users tend to mix hallucinogens with other drugs, such as marijuana and alcohol. Doing so can have an impact on the severity and content of the trip.

INACCURATE—All hallucinogens are derived from nature.

ACCURATE—While some hallucinogens, including psilocybin ('magic mushrooms'), DMT (dimethyltryptamine), Salvia divinorum, and mescaline (from the peyote cactus) can be found naturally, LSD, for example, is made synthetically. Synthetic hallucinogens are derived from phenethylamine, which is altered in a laboratory to create effects that mimic those of natural hallucinogens. The molecular structures of all phenethylamines contain a phenyl ring joined to an amino group via an ethyl side chain (phenyl-ethyl-amine).

INACCURATE—If you take any hallucinogen, you will trip for just a few hours.

ACCURATE—The "trip length" of a full dose of psychedelics can differ drastically based on which type of drug you ingest. LSD trips tend to be the longest, and while they typically range from six to eleven hours, some users have reported even longer trips lasting up to fourteen hours.

INACCURATE—LSD can damage your DNA.

ACCURATE—In recent years, several LSD clinical studies have examined the white blood cells of participants and have found no evidence that LSD can alter or damage DNA. However, more research needs to be done to determine the nature and severity of the effects.

INACCURATE—There are no long-lasting adverse effects from the continued use of hallucinogens.

ACCURATE—Neurological effects can range from mild to severe depending on the drug, the dose used, and the amount of time the drug is used.

INACCURATE—Hallucinogenic drugs make you more intelligent.

ACCURATE—Hallucinogenic drugs alter perceptions and information processing. They will create mental pictures that are vastly different from a person's typical neurological representation. However, no evidence suggests that they make you more intelligent.

INACCURATE—Hallucinogens can be used to treat a wide variety of personality disorders and other mental health concerns.

ACCURATE—The research indicates that hallucinogens can be used to treat conditions like post-traumatic stress disorder (PTSD), depression, and anxiety. However, significantly more research needs to be done to determine the long-term effects of continued use. Also, these drugs must be administered under the close supervision of qualified medical personnel.

MARIJUANA

INACCURATE—Smoking marijuana is more harmful than smoking cigarettes.

ACCURATE—Research suggests that smoking cannabis is generally less harmful than smoking tobacco. However, it is important to note that smoking marijuana can still negatively affect the heart and respiratory system.

INACCURATE—Marijuana is not considered to be addictive.

ACCURATE—Marijuana, just like any other drug, can be addictive. There seem to be fewer problems with occasional use, but when used daily, especially in users who use it several times per day, dependence on the drug does develop.

INACCURATE—Consuming edibles and vaping are safe ways to use marijuana.

ACCURATE—Whereas they may be safer than smoking the drug, they still affect the brain and nervous system. More research is needed to clarify the long-term effects.

INACCURATE—Marijuana is safe to use during pregnancy and breastfeeding.

ACCURATE—Marijuana is not recommended, even for medicinal purposes, during preconception, pregnancy, or lactation.

INACCURATE—It is safe to drive after smoking marijuana.

ACCURATE—Since marijuana is a central nervous system depressant, it can slow reaction times, and there are also concerns about maintaining one's attention while operating a motor vehicle.

INACCURATE—Marijuana helps one's mood and promotes mental health.

ACCURATE—There is research evidence to indicate that marijuana can have a positive effect on mood, especially as it relates to anxiety and mild depression. The second part of this statement is questionable. There is no evidence to suggest that marijuana promotes mental health. As a drug, it is designed to treat symptoms. Mental health treatment requires addressing the causes of those mental health problems.

INACCURATE—There are no long-term disadvantages to using marijuana.

ACCURATE—Aside from short-term memory problems, long-term effects include heart and cardiovascular problems, short-term memory issues, and focusing problems. Cannabinoid hyperemesis syndrome (CHS), a condition that leads to repeated and severe bouts of vomiting, has been reported. It is rare and only occurs in daily long-term users of marijuana. Also, there are issues regarding motivation and accountability with chronic use of marijuana.

INACCURATE—There are no advantages to using marijuana.

ACCURATE—Marijuana does have positive medicinal effects such as chronic pain reduction, relief of issues related to glaucoma, and reduction in anxiety and rumination. It also helps to relieve low-grade depression, ease muscle spasms, nausea, and vomiting, and increase appetite.

INACCURATE: Marijuana stays in your bloodstream for just a few days.

ACCURATE: Marijuana is fat soluble and remains in your body and your bloodstream for considerably longer than alcohol. It could remain as long as thirty days after its last use for daily users.

INACCURATE—Since marijuana is legalized in many states, it is safe to drive a motor vehicle when using it.

ACCURATE—While it is legal to use marijuana in many states, in most states, you can still be charged with a DUI if marijuana is found in your bloodstream

FOOD

INACCURATE—Food addiction doesn't exist.

ACCURATE—Food addiction is a viable addiction. It introduces many of the same neurological changes we see in other addictions.

INACCURATE—Anorexia and bulimia are not food addictions.

ACCURATE—Both Anorexia and bulimia are food addictions that can have disastrous consequences for those suffering from them.

INACCURATE—Food addiction culture is the same as diet culture.

ACCURATE—Diets are often used by people who want to look better, feel better, and be healthier. Food addictions are more psychologically based, and often, a person is struggling emotionally.

INACCURATE—Once someone develops a food addiction, they will always be addicted to food.

ACCURATE—Like any other addiction, there is recovery, and there are slips and movements backward. It is always important to have a program that helps you stay in recovery. Food addiction is no exception.

INACCURATE—Eating disorders are a matter of choice or lifestyle.

ACCURATE—No one chooses to have an eating disorder, but what often starts as a reasonable plan to "get healthy" or "fit" through diet and exercise can transform into an unhealthy and potentially life-threatening illness.

INACCURATE—Food addictions and eating disorders are often a way to control other people.

ACCURATE—At times, there is a control mechanism at work, but often, the person may feel out of control, and food may be used to help them feel that they have something to control in their life.

INACCURATE—If you have a food addiction, you also have an eating disorder.

ACCURATE—This isn't always true. Someone can have a food addiction and an eating disorder, but this is not always the case. Some people cannot stop consuming food, while others are using it for other mental health concerns.

INACCURATE—If you have a food addiction, you also have mental health concerns.

ACCURATE—Some people are merely addicted to the process of eating. You do not need to have mental health concerns to have a food addiction.

GAMBLING

INACCURATE—Gambling addiction is not a true addiction.

ACCURATE—Gambling causes the same neurological changes that we see in drug addiction. It causes changes at the physical and neurological levels.

INACCURATE—Every gambler gambles for the big payday.

ACCURATE—Most gambling addicts talk about the big payday, but the real reason to gamble is the rush that comes from playing the game.

INACCURATE—Gamblers can walk away if they are winning.

ACCURATE—Staying in the game is very much like what happens when a drug addict is using. For some people, it is almost impossible to leave the game.

INACCURATE—12-step programs do not help people with gambling addictions.

ACCURATE—12-step programs can be quite beneficial in helping people with gambling addictions.

INACCURATE—Teenagers cannot develop gambling addictions.

ACCURATE—Just as with any other addiction, age is not always a factor. Young people can become addicted to gambling.

INACCURATE—Becoming knowledgeable about how to play the game will make you a better gambler and help you avoid gambling addiction.

ACCURATE—It doesn't matter how much you know about the game. Once a person is in the game, the addiction can take over, and rational thinking all but disappears.

INACCURATE—Once you develop a gambling addiction, you will always be addicted to gambling.

ACCURATE—Just like with any other addiction, you can still fall prey to the active addictive process, but there is also a way to enter recovery. If you continue to work with your recovery program, there is a good chance of staying in recovery.

SMARTPHONES AND OTHER ELECTRONIC DEVICES

INACCURATE—Technology is not a drug.

ACCURATE—Overusing technology produces the same neurological effects as other addictions.

INACCURATE—There is no withdrawal from not using your smartphone or electronic games.

ACCURATE—There is certainly a withdrawal. Usually, it begins with "reasons to check the smartphone," followed by the emergency instigating the need to use it. After approximately twelve hours without using a smartphone, many people become agitated, short-tempered, and angry. The same rules apply to gamers.

INACCURATE—People's lives don't drastically change when they stop using smartphones and other forms of technology.

ACCURATE—People feel disconnected when they stop using their smartphones, laptops, games, etc. This feeling exacerbates the addictive process. When people avoid their smartphones and other electronics for a significant amount of time, say two weeks, they often report greater life stability, clearer perspective, and improvements in their communication and personal relationships.

INACCURATE—There is no research to back up the notion of smartphone addiction.

ACCURATE—Research does support the addictive processes associated with smartphone overuse. One study observed increased anxiety and emotional arousal in participants deprived of their smartphones.

INACCURATE—People are usually honest and straightforward about their smartphone and gaming use.

ACCURATE—People use the same deceit and defense mechanisms with smartphones and gaming addictions that we see in other forms of addiction.

INACCURATE—Overusing smartphones and video games does not interfere with relationships and family life.

ACCURATE—Both addictions cause one to isolate and reduce communication and the working relationship that comes from family and social interaction.

INACCURATE—Smartphones increase social interaction with other people.

ACCURATE—The amount of interaction with others is increased, but the quality of the interaction tends to decrease. Face-to-face contact is always the best for quality communication. Overusing texting provides more interaction time but does not provide the quality of communication that comes with close physical contact.

INACCURATE—Smartphone addiction is typically relegated to younger people, such as teenagers and college students.

ACCURATE—Like any other addiction, smartphone addiction knows no age, gender, socioeconomic status, etc. Adults are just as likely to become addicted to smartphone use as their younger counterparts.

SEX AND PORNOGRAPHY

INACCURATE—Sex is natural and is not an addiction.

ACCURATE—The first part of the statement is accurate. However, sex addiction and viewing pornography can provide the same neurological stimulation as drugs and alcohol and can develop into addictions.

INACCURATE—Sex addictions don't hurt anyone else.

ACCURATE—Sex addiction and viewing pornography addictions can have a dramatic impact on relationships and family dynamics.

INACCURATE—There are no lasting consequences from viewing pornographic material regularly.

ACCURATE—Occasional viewing of pornographic material shows no lingering effects. However, routine indulgence can cause guilt, shame, and secrecy.

INACCURATE—Sex addiction and pornography do not affect healthy sexual relationships.

ACCURATE—For some people, sex addictions can lead to extramarital relationships, dissatisfaction with sexual contact from one's significant other, and distance in an intimate relationship. Pornography, for some people, is a replacement for healthy sexual relationships, especially when viewed alone and without one's significant other. Pornography can also instigate expectations that often cannot be fulfilled in a healthy sexual relationship.

INACCURATE—Sex and pornography addictions are related to fetishes and other dysfunctional sexual dynamics.

ACCURATE—A sex addiction is an obsession with sex, while viewing pornography has more to do with voyeurism and satisfying sexual urges. They are not all associated with fetishes and other dysfunctional sexual dynamics.

INACCURATE—Sex and pornography addictions are primarily a male thing.

ACCURATE—Whereas men tend to engage in these addictions more often than women, women are just as susceptible to them as their male counterparts.

INACCURATE—There is no recovery from sex and pornography addictions.

ACCURATE—Recovery can be difficult; however, programs are available to help people recover. Also, counseling with sex and pornography addicts is highly successful, provided the counseling services are offered by someone who understands the dynamics and recovery methods that are needed and that the addicted person continues with the treatment until successful discharge from the counseling program.

SELF-HARM

INACCURATE—Self-harm is a suicide attempt.

ACCURATE—Self-harm can occur without suicidal ideation.

INACCURATE—Cutting is the only form of self-harm.

ACCURATE—Cutting is a common form of self-harm, but there are other types of self-harming behavior. Some individuals who self-harm may burn themselves, pull their hair, scratch themselves, break bones, or bang their heads.

INACCURATE—Self-harm is extremely rare.

ACCURATE—Rates of self-harm are higher than most people realize. Very few people report that they harm themselves, so obtaining accurate statistics can be difficult.

INACCURATE—Self-harm is an attention-seeking behavior.

ACCURATE—Individuals who self-harm are typically ashamed of their behavior and want to hide it.

INACCURATE—People who self-injure do not feel pain.

ACCURATE—People who engage in self-harming behavior do feel pain, but they may experience it differently than those who do not self-harm. Their bodies and minds adjust to the continuous harm, and their brains can interpret it as pleasureful as it causes them to feel less pain from other sources.

INACCURATE—People self-injure as a way to manipulate others.

ACCURATE—Self-harm is not intended to be an act of manipulation. Self-harm is typically used for stress relief and diversion from emotional pain.

INACCURATE—Individuals who self-harm have been abused.

ACCURATE—Having a history of abuse can increase the risk of self-harm, but not everyone who self-injures has been abused. Pain can come from other sources, such as family dysfunction, bullying, substance abuse, and body image.

INACCURATE—Self-harm is just a phase that teens will outgrow.

ACCURATE—Self-harm is a serious concern that requires intervention. The issues that lead to self-harm can be complicated, and counseling programs are strongly suggested.

INACCURATE—Most people do not recover from self-abuse addiction.

ACCURATE—As with any addiction, there may be an urge to continue with the behavior. However, counseling programs are very successful in bringing people to and helping them maintain recovery. It can be an involved process, but if the person stays with the program, the results are usually good.

SHOPPING

INACCURATE—There is no such thing as shopping addiction.

ACCURATE—Addiction to shopping and the acquisition process can develop into an obsessive-compulsive condition and a full-blown addiction.

INACCURATE—Emotions have nothing to do with compulsive shopping.

ACCURATE—When someone is addicted to shopping, they may experience a sense of euphoria or excitement when they shop, followed by feelings of regret or guilt. The emotional experience related to shopping is what fuels the addiction. There may also be emotional motivators that lead to the compulsion.

INACCURATE—People with shopping problems can easily stop by simply not going shopping.

ACCURATE—When addicted to shopping, individuals will continue to shop even though they know it negatively affects their lives. They will feel an uncontrolled desire to keep shopping or make purchases despite any adverse consequences that occur because of it. They may do this by physically visiting stores or by shopping online.

INACCURATE—People shop because they like to acquire new things.

ACCURATE—Very often, the products shopaholics buy are not used. It is the process of shopping, similar to what we see with gamblers, that creates the addiction and helps maintain it.

INACCURATE—Once an individual finishes a shopping spree, they feel relief and don't want to shop for a while.

ACCURATE—People with shopping addictions think about shopping often. This does not always stop when the shopping spree is over.

INACCURATE—Shopping is a selfish behavior and is not connected to mental health issues.

ACCURATE—Shopping may become a coping tool for dealing with stress, anxiety, or other negative feelings. Individuals may also experience decreased feelings of depression when shopping, as well as emotional distress or a sense of emptiness when not shopping.

INACCURATE—People with shopping addictions are truthful about what they are doing.

ACCURATE—Individuals may hide their shopping habits from others, feeling shame or embarrassment about their compulsive purchases. For instance, a person may wait until their spouse is asleep before bringing in purchases from the car to hide them in the closet before they notice what they've bought.

INACCURATE—Addictive shopping is something people do in their spare time.

ACCURATE—Shopping may replace other essential responsibilities, such as work, school, or family obligations. Excessive shopping may cause individuals to ignore their loved ones, their self-care or health, and their work responsibilities.

INACCURATE—Addicted shoppers will stop shopping when their money runs out.

ACCURATE—Once an addicted shopper has used up all their resources due to a shopping addiction, they may want to shoplift or attempt to open credit cards in family member's names just to get funds to shop.

WORKAHOLISM

INACCURATE—Workaholism is not a true addiction.

ACCURATE—Addiction to work shows many of the physical and neurological components we see with other addictions.

INACCURATE—Work addiction is a product of a commitment to the job and their colleagues.

ACCURATE—Though workaholics tend to be loyal to the company they work for, they exhibit these obsessive-compulsive traits in other areas of their lives, such as working around the house and working for volunteer organizations.

INACCURATE—Workaholism is primarily an adult disorder.

ACCURATE—Though we see the symptoms manifest in adulthood, workaholism starts much earlier. It can be seen in the high school years by students who overindulge in studies, part-time jobs, and other work-related functions.

INACCURATE—Workaholism can be a positive thing.

ACCURATE—The positives associated with workaholism are usually relegated to efficient job performance and enhanced finances. However, consistent with any other addiction, it causes problems in other areas, such as relationships, responsibilities at home, and personal commitments.

INACCURATE—Workaholism is primarily a mental health concern.

ACCURATE—Workaholism is an obsessive-compulsive trait that affects a person's body and emotions. Workaholics often have poor sleep habits and either skip meals or eat unhealthy foods when they are working.

Emotionally, they tend to be more reactive and defensive, especially about the time they spend at work.

INACCURATE—Workaholics have more energy. This is why they indulge in work-related activities with intensity.

ACCURATE—While there is truth that one does need more energy to accomplish the tasks a workaholic endeavors to complete, they are typically obsessive-compulsive and often type A personalities, that is, people who are intense and want their world to be ordered and accurate.

INACCURATE—A job that never ends or requires long hours and includes work that needs to be taken home is what creates a workaholic.

ACCURATE—Most people balk at working longer hours and taking work home. Workaholics not only accept these challenges, but they also actively seek them.

INACCURATE—The only reason workaholics work is because the work needs to be done.

ACCURATE-Workaholics often work to avoid emotional difficulties, past problems, or current issues in their lives, such as relationships, financial problems, or personal loss.

INACCURATE—A workaholic will always be a workaholic.

ACCURATE—With intervention and counseling, Workaholics can learn to set boundaries and view work-related functions realistically. Counseling will also help them address issues they may have been avoiding by overloading their schedules with work.

EXERCISE

INACCURATE—Exercising cannot develop into an addiction.

ACCURATE—Exercising can increase the production of chemicals like dopamine and endorphins. Because these have a pleasurable effect on the brain, intense exercise over a long period can become habit-forming and develop into an addiction.

INACCURATE—The more you exercise, the healthier you will be.

ACCURATE—The body needs rest periods to rejuvenate and repair muscles that become damaged during exercise. Moderate exercise followed by rest is the healthiest formula.

INACCURATE—People always exercise to become healthier.

ACCURATE—For some people, body image is an issue. Regardless of how healthy they become, they never seem to be happy with their progress.

INACCURATE—Body image always gets better with continued exercise.

ACCURATE—For some people, the more they work out, the more they obsess about their body image. This is the fuel that feeds the addiction since they will work harder and longer to achieve the ideal body.

INACCURATE—Runner's high is simply a temporary euphoric state that develops while someone is running.

ACCURATE—While this is true, runner's high extends beyond the running period. A person who develops runner's high can withdraw if they don't routinely run. This usually develops among long-distance runners.

INACCURATE—The more you exercise, the better the results.

ACCURATE—Exercise must be followed by rest. Addictive exercisers tend to overexercise, and after some time, they will begin to see muscle loss because overexercising does not give muscles enough time to rest.

INACCURATE—Exercising is positive and doesn't cause other problems in a person's life.

ACCURATE—Exercise addicts can spend a long time in the gym. In addition to some physical problems that can develop, the addiction can consume their lives, and relationships and other responsibilities tend to fall by the wayside.

INACCURATE—If a person realizes they have become addicted to exercise, all they need to do is adjust their workout schedule.

ACCURATE—Since exercise causes chemical changes in the brain, readjusting the schedule is difficult. Exercise addicts have a difficult time keeping their workouts and workout times in a healthy perspective.

INACCURATE—If an exercise addict attempts to change their schedule, they will lose the benefits of their intense program and become unhappy people.

ACCURATE—The human body operates according to specific physical laws. When exercise addicts understand the healthy parameters they need to apply to their workouts, the gains are often increased. As they change their schedule, there will be a period of discomfort. However, their brains will adjust, and their lives will generally become happier and more productive.

SUMMING IT UP

As you can see, addiction stretches far beyond the boundaries of drugs and alcohol. Though any addiction will change neurotransmitter production in the brain, the application of that change depends on the type of addiction and how deep into the addiction a person has gone. Often, we will see people involved in several addictions, or they may replace one addiction with another. I will discuss this further as we proceed.

For now, you need to become knowledgeable about the various types of addiction, how they develop, how they continue to manifest, and what you can do to address them. This chapter presented some of the basic facts of the addictions covered in this book. Though the list is not exhaustive, it does represent the more typical types of addiction that people experience.

Regardless of the type of addiction you have, they all tend to be subject to the same parameters. Physical and neurological functioning changes; people lose intellectual perspective regarding the healthy use of a substance or activity and emotionally become defensive when those parameters are challenged. It doesn't matter what you are addicted to or why. Addiction always results in a loss of control and collateral damage to your life and the lives of those close to you.

If you or someone close to you is experiencing any of the addictions listed above, it is good to know as much as you can about it. If there is an addiction you are experiencing that is not mentioned in this chapter, it makes good sense to begin acquiring the facts that define it. No one has to be an active addict for their entire life. There is *always* help. Acquiring the facts begins the process.

 TIME TO TAKE ACTION

1. Be willing to take an honest look at addiction and how it may be affecting your life and those close to you.

2. Review the facts related to the specific types of addiction and ask yourself if any of them pertain to you or someone close to you.

3. Make a list of those facts that you or someone close to you may be experiencing.

4. Enlist the health of someone close to you or an addiction professional to help you understand the depth and breadth of any addiction that may be affecting your life or that of someone close to you.

 DRIVING IT HOME

This chapter provided specific information about various types of addiction and how they develop. Don't try to make any decisions just yet. You are in the information-gathering stage. As we move on, I will present information in greater detail regarding each type of addiction. I will provide specific information to assist you in each chapter, and in Chapters 19 through 30, I will help you establish a treatment plan to address your addiction or the addiction of someone close to you.

YOUR DECLARATION IS: *I will get the facts to understand and gain control over my addiction!*

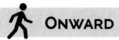 **ONWARD**

In the next chapter, I will examine alcohol as a normal way of life for so many people. I will discuss the excuses people use to drink, how the abuse and addictive cycle develops, the defense mechanisms people use to deny its significance in their lives, and the damage it is causing to them and their loved ones. I will also present the steps necessary to help address this menacing addiction.

CHAPTER 3

Alcohol—Deniably So

It's the great trickster. As it lulls you into complacency, it can change your world forever.

PROCESSES TO EMPLOY: Brutal Honesty, I Over E, Present-Understand-Fix, Slowing Down Life's Pace, Internal Focus, Fact-Finding, Honesty, Patience, Truth-Telling, Belief, Listening, Trust

---

NO OTHER DRUG IN HUMAN EXISTENCE has been used more often than alcohol. It is the easiest drug to produce and is used for virtually every occasion, from funerals to weddings, as well as for small gatherings and personal pleasure. Alcohol is used as a reward for a day's hard work, to reduce stress, to escape worry, and to relax. Its use spans the planet and has survived prohibitions and attacks from legal entities and special interest groups.

THE STATISTICS

Here are recent statistics regarding alcohol:[2]

1. Over 138 million Americans aged twelve and over drink alcohol, and over 28 million, or 20.4% of them, have a problem with alcohol.

2. The rate of all alcohol-related ER visits increased 47 percent between 2006 and 2014, which translates to an average annual increase of 210,000 alcohol-related emergency visits.

3. Alcohol contributes to about 18.5 percent of emergency room visits and 22.1 percent of overdose deaths related to prescription opioids.

4. An estimated 95,000 people (approximately 68,000 men and 27,000 women) die from alcohol-related causes annually, making alcohol the third-leading preventable cause of death in the United States.

5. Between 2011 and 2015, the leading causes of alcohol-attributable deaths due to chronic conditions in the United States were alcohol-associated liver disease, heart disease and stroke, unspecified liver cirrhosis, upper aerodigestive tract cancers, liver cancer, supraventricular cardiac dysrhythmia, alcohol-attributable deaths, breast cancer, and hypertension.

6. In 2015, alcohol-impaired driving fatalities accounted for 10,265 deaths (29 percent of overall driving fatalities).

I define an "alcohol problem" as *the use of alcohol to the point that it causes physical problems, emotional issues, legal problems, financial concerns, and/or family and relationship issues. I am describing alcoholism as the inability to control drinking due to both a physical and emotional dependence on alcohol.* Alcoholism has been described as a disease, though the support for this description is not as strong as it was twenty years ago.

THE PROGRESSION

Though there are genetic predispositions to alcohol abuse and alcoholism, no one is born an *active* alcoholic. Once introduced to the substance, some people will walk away from it, some will incorporate it into their lives on weekends and special occasions, some will use small amounts daily to relax, and some will have difficulty separating themselves from it.

For those who may have a difficult time keeping their alcohol use in perspective, there is often a slow but steady progression as the dependence develops. Very rarely does the dependence on a substance show itself immediately. There are always steps that one progresses through until addiction is realized. The progression from initial use to the point of dependence and addiction are:

1. The person uses alcohol for the first time and finds its effects soothing or intriguing.

2. During later social occasions, alcohol is consumed again, and the mind begins to adjust to the euphoria the alcohol produces.

3. In subsequent drinking episodes, to produce enhanced euphoria, more alcohol is consumed.

4. As alcohol consumption continues, both the amount of alcohol and the number of times spent consuming it increases.

5. There may be experimentation with different kinds of alcohol both to widen one's drinking experiences and to determine which types of alcohol produce the best euphoric feelings.

6. Time and resources are beginning to be set aside to ensure that alcohol and alcohol-related situations remain available.

7. Even with no special events scheduled, alcohol is consumed simply for the experience.

8. Drinking begins to occur alone, at home, usually to relax at the end of the day.

9. Larger amounts of alcohol are consumed alone, and alcohol is kept in the house "just in case visitors come."

10. Alcohol is now being consumed regularly, as defined by personal needs.

11. Excuses are made to continue drinking alcohol, and the person is minimizing their use and beginning to lie about the amount being consumed.

12. Alcohol-related problems are beginning to affect the person's health, relationships, family interactions, finances, or other responsibilities.

13. In more advanced cases, the addict may experience personality changes, and in drastic cases, significant physical problems such as liver, heart, and brain damage may occur.

Not everyone works the steps the same way. In some cases, steps may be skipped, and the progression from the person's initial use of the drink to the point of addiction occurs faster. In other cases, progressionthrough each step is slower. In yet other cases more time is spent on the initial steps with an increase of speed at the end. Once a person progresses to the point of alcoholism, their lives will drastically change for the worse.

IN THE CLUTCHES

When alcoholism takes over someone's life, everything about their life will change in some form. It will affect their relationships, employment, family life, social life, personal health, personality, and temperament. When this begins to happen, the alcoholic will employ a system of defense mechanisms designed to hide the severity of the problem from others and to defend the continued use of alcohol. A list of the defense mechanisms addicts use are:

➤ **Denial**—the refusal to accept behaving as if a painful event, thought, or feeling does not exist.

➤ **Projection**—assigning undesired thoughts, feelings, or impulses to another person.

➤ **Intellectualization**—making something sound more important than it is or providing what seems like an intelligent reason for doing something.

➤ **Rationalization**—attempting to explain or justify one's behavior or attitude with logical, plausible reasons, even when these are not true or appropriate.

➤ **Sublimation**—modifying the natural expression of an inappropriate behavior to one that is socially acceptable.

➤ **Compensation**—overachieving in one area to compensate for short-comings in another.

➤ **Diversion**—attempting to move attention away from an event or behavior to something that has nothing to do with what is happening.

When alcohol takes over someone's life, they will be unreceptive to other people's concerns, complaints, and advice. Loved ones may raise concerns about the amount of time and money spent on alcohol. They may complain about responsibilities left unattended, financial problems, and relationship issues. They may offer advice for improving the alcoholic's health, which can be at risk while in the grasp of alcoholism. Anything along these lines can be perceived as a threat to the continued use of the drug, and an alcoholic will do whatever is necessary to fend off these perceived assaults, which are usually attempts to help and not assaults at all.

IN THE CLUTCHES

Look for the following changes in yourself or in the person you care about who is drinking. These problems and issues indicate that alcohol consumption has become a full-blown addiction:

PHYSICAL PROBLEMS—Alcohol is one of those drugs that causes a wide array of physical problems. *The brain:* Alcohol interferes with the brain's communication pathways and can affect the way the brain looks and works. These disruptions can change mood and behavior, making it harder to think clearly and move with coordination. *The heart:* Dangers to the heart include cardiomyopathy (stretching and drooping of heart muscle), arrhythmias(irregular heartbeat), stroke, and high blood pressure. *The liver:* Heavy drinking takes a toll on the liver and can lead to a variety of problems and liver inflammation, including steatosis or fatty liver, alcoholic hepatitis, fibrosis, and cirrhosis. *The pancreas:* Pancreatitis is a painful and potentially fatal inflammation of the pancreas. *Cancer:* Drinking alcohol increases the risk of cancers, including esophageal cancer, liver cancer, breast cancer, and colorectal cancer.

MENTAL HEALTH ISSUES—Alcohol decelerates how fast the brain processes information, making it harder to understand one's feelings and the possible consequences of one's actions. The chemical changes in the brain can soon lead to frequent negative emotions, anger, depression, and/or anxiety.

COMMUNICATION PROBLEMS—Since alcohol interferes with the brain's communication pathways and can affect how the brain works, it makes it harder for the brain areas that control balance, memory, and speech, all of which affect efficient communication, to operate efficiently. It also makes it more difficult to retrieve information and put it in a proper perspective to be communicated.

LEGAL PROBLEMS—Drunk driving, arrests, court-ordered treatment, fines, jail time, job loss, and other legal consequences can all result from overconsuming alcohol. People generally drink to have fun, but this can quickly turn into overdrinking and bad decisions with long-term consequences.

FINANCIAL CONCERNS—The financial consequences of alcoholism can be severe, particularly for those who already have financial limitations. Apart from the money spent on drinks, alcoholics may suffer other financial problems such as lower wages and lost employment opportunities, increased medical and legal expenses, decreased eligibility for loans, and late payments.

FAMILY AND RELATIONSHIP ISSUES—Chronic alcohol use alters both mood and inhibitions, affecting decision-making in the moment, meaning an individual is more likely to make rash choices or perhaps instigate verbal or physical confrontations that they later regret. In addition, problematic alcohol use and alcoholism can strain relationships with family members, friends, and others. At the extreme, heavy drinking can contribute to domestic violence and child abuse or neglect. Alcohol use is often involved when people become violent, as well as when they are violently attacked.

EMPLOYMENT PROBLEMS—Absenteeism is estimated to be four to eight times greater among alcoholics and alcohol abusers (those who abuse alcohol but are not addicted to it). Other family members of alcoholics also have greater rates of absenteeism as they attempt to address situations that arise due to the alcoholic's behavior. Accidents and on-the-job injuries are far more prevalent among alcoholics and alcohol abusers. They are also more argumentative. Alcoholism in the workplace can be extremely costly to an employer. Drinking not only increases the possibility of employees getting injured, but it can also lead to more on-the-job accidents. Additionally, alcohol can cause a lack of concentration and coordination in an employee's work performance.

CHANGES IN SOCIAL LIFE—Alcoholics tend to be more argumentative. They react quickly and tend to have poor filters, often insulting and embarrassing those around them. In addition, their behavior is often questionable. They may act out, make themselves look foolish, and be aggressive or violent toward others.

LYING—Anytime someone is covering or defending an addiction, there will be difficulties telling the truth. Alcoholics not only lie about their drinking, but they will also evade the truth about everyday things as often as they can. This is used as a control device as they attempt to keep others off balance as much as possible.

ACCOUNTABILITY ISSUES—Alcoholics like to do what they want to do when they want to do it. They don't like being told what to do and have difficulty following orders. Often, their responsibilities at home, work, and to others are either poorly addressed or not addressed at all.

PERSONALITY CHANGES—Alcohol is often seen as a social lubricant. Some people do become more social. However, the quality of their social interactions is severely affected by the drug and not seen as healthy. Conversely, some people will become more introverted when they drink. Other concerns are effects on conscientiousness, openness, agreeableness, ambition, creativity, confidence, compassion, and curiosity.

ANGER AND VIOLENCE—Alcohol affects perceptions, deductive reasoning, and the ability to work through emotional situations rationally. Alcoholics often enter into reactive violent situations and, at times, will provoke people to create aggressive situations. Sometimes, the violence remains at the verbal level, but it can escalate into an unprovoked physical attack.

Not everyone experiences alcoholism and the problems it creates in the same way. Some people may experience many of the changes just discussed. Others may experience only a few. The intensity and duration can also differ from person to person. Regardless, chronic and sustained abuse of alcohol does change one's life, and the changes are rarely, if ever, positive.

COLLATERAL DAMAGE

There is no limit to the amount of damage alcoholism can cause in an alcoholic's life. Alcoholics believe that any physical problems their addiction causes are something only they need to deal with. However, the family must also deal with physical problems since they may be involved in surgeries, doctor visits, caretaking, and recuperation times. As the alcoholic's mental health deteriorates, resulting in depression, anxiety, or any other personality changes, those close to them are also affected, and communication begins to break down. Either there will be a complete lack of communication or the alcoholic may be abusive and degrading at times.

When the alcoholic misses work, overspends to purchase alcohol, or spends time and money at the bar, family members suffer from the reduction in finances. Legal problems will further drain the finances, and family members are always part of the legal process. This could be in the form of meetings with attorneys, court appearances, trying to keep things going when the alcoholic is incarcerated, and the financial drain from the entire legal process. All of this can severely impact family life, health, and relationships.

Alcoholics often miss time at work or may lose jobs due to poor performance, absenteeism, or tardiness. Also, their relationships with work associates can suffer, leading to suspensions and, at times, dismissal. All too often, the family's social life changes since the alcoholic either withdraws from social events, makes a fool of themselves during these events, or destroys relationships at the hands of the addiction. All through the process, the alcoholic will be defensive and lie about what they are doing. This puts a further strain on family relationships as the alcoholic continues to attempt to hide their problem from the rest of the family.

As the condition progresses, the family experiences a sharp reduction in accountability. Alcoholics will say they are going to do something, attend an event, or take care of their responsibilities. Still, often, they do not hold themselves accountable and fail to take care of their commitments. As their personality changes, they may become vindictive, argumentative, and verbally abusive. In severe cases, they may become angry people, and it's not uncommon for violence to become part of the picture. Unfortunately, family members are on the receiving end of the alcoholic's abuse.

SUMMING IT UP

All addictions cause collateral damage. Even if the alcoholic lives alone, people on the periphery (i.e., extended family, relatives, and close friends) might experience collateral damage. Also, collateral damage can refer to the changes listed earlier. As I am using it, "collateral" means *additional but subordinate; secondary.* In the case of alcoholism, alcohol abuse is the primary condition. All other conditions, whether they pertain to family members and friends or factors like legal problems, financial concerns, and social communication problems, are secondary to the primary problem. They are created by alcoholism and are intertwined with it. They affect the way the alcoholic lives life, thereby affecting the lives of everyone close to them.

Whether you are an active alcoholic or a family member of an alcoholic, it is important to take stock of what is occurring in your life as a result of alcoholism. You can do this by referring to the list above and determining which of the issues have an impact on your life. If several of these are problematic for you, it is time to consider getting help. Alcohol is a drug, and drugs *do* affect the way people live. Take stock of the conditions affecting your life.

If you need help, you can call the alcohol emergency hotline at 1 (800) 662-HELP (4357). Everything is confidential.

⏱ TIME TO TAKE ACTION

1. This is the time to start being honest with yourself. Whether you are the person drinking or it's someone close to you, nothing changes until you get honest with yourself. Make this your first decision.

2. Make a list of all the ways alcohol may be negatively impacting your life.

3. Review the list of items affecting your life and discuss each with a friend or other trusted individual. This will help you understand what is affecting you and how deep the problem goes.

4. People often hide alcoholism, whether it's their issue or a family member's. If you believe alcoholism is having a negative impact on your life, talk about it with someone close to you. It's always good to accept support from others as you begin to address this problem.

5. It is essential to enlist the services of a professional counselor. This should be someone well versed not only in personal and family members but also in the dynamics and treatment of addiction.

6. If you think you cannot stop drinking or if you have tried and have been unable to do so, you may be an alcoholic. Consider going to your first Alcoholics Anonymous meeting. These people understand what you are experiencing, have been there, and know how to help you address the problem.

7. If you believe a loved one is an alcoholic and you could use some support from others, consider going to an Al-Anon meeting. This organization addresses the needs of those whom someone else's alcoholism has impacted. You can find meeting lists in your area online.

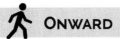

DRIVING IT HOME

Alcohol is indeed a drug, and like any drug, it can have a devastating impact on the lives of the alcoholic and those close to them. Alcoholism has the power to change every aspect of one's life and the lives of those close to them. There is a fine line between social drinking and problematic drinking. That line is often blurred by fear and defensive thoughts and behaviors. Nothing changes until you become honest about what is happening in your life at the hands of alcoholism. Be willing to take stock of what is happening to you and those close to you. Enlist the help of others to give you a more accurate perspective and be willing to get the help you need from professionals and other support people. Alcoholism can be devastating, but its effects do not have to be permanent.

YOUR DECLARATION IS: *I will get honest with myself, and I will begin to address the problems alcohol is causing for me and my family!*

ONWARD

Smoking is another addiction that has been with us for centuries. In the next chapter, I will examine nicotine's effect on the smoker's life and those close to them. I will also address vaping nicotine, which has become a popular alternative to smoking cigarettes, but certainly not a healthy one. I will examine the effects nicotine addiction has on one's family and how to address this powerful addiction.

◇◇◇◇◇◇◇◇◇◇◇◇

CHAPTER 4

Nicotine—Empty Promises

Smoking adds nothing to your life, and in the end, it takes your breath away.

PROCESSES TO EMPLOY: Brutal Honesty, I Over E, Slowing Down Life's Pace, Internal Focus, Fact-Finding, Honesty, Patience, Truth-Telling, Belief, Listening, Trust

---

SMOKING OFTEN BEGINS AS A WAY TO LOOK COOL, to fit in with the crowd, to rebel, or to make a social statement. It provides no euphoria, adds no quality to anyone's life, can be a dirty and offensive habit, and has become quite expensive. For most people, smoking begins in adolescence, but that isn't always the case. Some people start as early as junior high school, while others never pick up a cigarette until they reach adulthood.

Usually, the first puff or drag on a cigarette quickly causes one to feel as though they are choking and gasping for breath. In addition, their heartbeat increases drastically, there is a feeling of lightheadedness, and one's eyes can burn profusely. However, habit formation, the brain's way of turning unhealthy decisions into new comfort zones, sets in, the brain and the body adjust to this toxic behavior, and the adverse reactions seem to disappear. It doesn't take long for the habit to continue and subsequently for the addiction to begin.

THE STATISTICS

Here are recent statistics regarding nicotine:[3]

➤ 57.277 million people use tobacco or nicotine products (vape).

- In 2021, 11.5% of U.S. adults (an estimated 28.3 million people) currently smoked cigarettes: 13.1% of men, 10.1% of women.

- In 2023, of those youth who ever tried e-cigarettes or vaping, approximately half reported currently using them, indicating that many youths who try e-cigarettes remain e-cigarette users.

- 57.277 million people use tobacco or nicotine products (vape).

Since the laws regulating smoking in public places have become stricter, there has been a slight decline in the use of tobacco; however, the use of nicotine has increased with the popularity of vaping. Today, it is easy to buy the cartridges used in vaping pens. Other people and businesses do not react to vaping the same way they did to cigarettes and cigars. Unfortunately, people are under the misconception that vaping is a healthier way to put nicotine into their bodies. Nicotine is still addictive in this form, and there are still side effects associated with its use. Among those side effects are dizziness and lightheadedness, sleep disturbances, changes in blood flow, headaches, increased risk of blood clotting, higher blood pressure, changes in heart rhythm and rate, and shortness of breath. So, one may change the delivery of the drug, but the adverse effects on the body remain.

Cigarette smoking leads to disease and disability and can affect nearly every organ of the body. Cigarette smoking remains the leading cause of preventable disease, disability, and death in the United States. The tobacco industry spends billions of dollars each year on marketing cigarettes. Smoking costs the United States hundreds of billions of dollars each year. Some of the ingredients in cigarettes include:

- **NICOTINE**—A colorless, poisonous alkaloid derived from the tobacco plant. It is a powerful drug that affects the brain and quickly becomes addictive.

- **TAR**—A sticky brown, toxic substance that forms when tobacco cools and condenses. It collects in the arteries and the lungs and can cause cancer.

➤ **CARBON MONOXIDE**—An odorless, colorless gas released from burning tobacco. When inhaled, it enters the bloodstream and interferes with the function of the heart and blood vessels. Up to 15 percent of a smoker's blood may contain carbon monoxide instead of oxygen.

➤ **ARSENIC**—A naturally occurring poisonous substance commonly used in rat poison. Arsenic occurs in small quantities in tobacco due to the arsenic-containing pesticides used in tobacco farming. Arsenic is commonly found in rat poison.

➤ **AMMONIA**—A toxic, colorless gas with a sharp odor. Ammonia compounds are commonly used in cleaning products and fertilizers. It is used to boost the impact of nicotine in manufactured cigarettes.

➤ **ACETONE**—A fragrant volatile liquid ketone, used as a solvent. Nail polish uses this solvent, for example.

➤ **TOLUENE**–A highly toxic chemical. Its industrial uses include rubbers, oils, resins, adhesives, inks, detergents, dyes, and explosives.

➤ **METHYLAMINE**–A chemical found in tanning lotion that is also used to make pharmaceuticals, insecticides, paint removers, surfactants, and rubber chemicals.

➤ **PESTICIDES**—Toxic chemicals used to kill pests, usually insects. These pesticides find their way into cigarettes because they are used in tobacco farming.

➤ **POLONIUM-210**—A radioactive element used in nuclear weapons and atomic heat sources. Called the perfect poison, it is a product of the radioactive decay of uranium-238, which decays to radon-222 and then to polonium. Polonium-210 has a half-life of 138 days.

➤ **METHANOL**—A toxic alcohol used industrially as a solvent, pesticide, and alternative fuel source. It is also a fuel source used in the aviation industry.

THE PROGRESSION

1. The prospective smoker becomes enamored with cigarette smoking as a way to fit in or rebel.

2. The prospective smoker will take a drag from someone else's cigarette to see what it feels like to smoke.

3. The smoker's body initially rejects the smoke and reacts with coughing, watering eyes, and lightheadedness, but the addictive properties of the nicotine cause them to use it again.

4. The smoker adjusts to the reaction by taking shallower breaths to mitigate the physical responses. They continue using this strategy until their body adapts and the aversive reactions disappear.

5. The prospective smoker lights up their own cigarette for the first time.

6. The smoker begins buying cigarettes.

7. The smoker now begins to smoke a cigarette several times a day.

8. In social situations, the smoker lights up more often. They also spend more time with other smokers.

9. The smoker stops hiding cigarettes and is more comfortable smoking in social situations.

10. The smoker graduates from social smoking to smoking alone.

11. The smoker begins to identify special times to smoke and begins to smoke "ritual" cigarettes. Examples of ritual smoking are smoking with a cup of coffee, after meals, with a glass of wine, or while reading the newspaper.

12. The smoker increases the number of cigarettes smoked per day.

13. The smoker begins to deny being addicted to cigarettes but understands that quitting could be difficult.

14. The smoker surrenders their defenses and admits they are addicted to nicotine.

As with all drugs, no one is immediately addicted to nicotine after the initial use. Though the steps of the progression may differ from person to person, there is always a progression. When a person does become addicted to nicotine, like any other drug, they will do what they need to do to secure the drug. It is not uncommon for smokers to leave the house in inclement weather to get a pack of cigarettes or a vape cartridge. If they run low on funds to purchase cigarettes, they will borrow money and, if necessary, steal it. At this point, smoking has become a dominating force in their lives.

IN THE CLUTCHES

The way nicotine is used has been changing in the last five years. There's been a shift from smoking cigarettes to vaping as a way to continue the nicotine addiction without the more harmful effects that come with smoking cigarettes. There is a misconception that vaping is a healthy way to acquire nicotine. There may be fewer adverse effects on one's health compared to smoking cigarettes, but vaping is not without health risks and has not been thoroughly studied over the long term. Vapor, like smoke, was never meant to routinely enter the lungs. It interferes with respiration and increases heart rate. Also, vaping liquid is not without additives. The commercial goal is for those who vape to become addicted and stay addicted.

Though nicotine addiction does not cause as many problems as other addictions, some of the problems it causes are considerably more potent. It is important to keep in mind that there is no such thing as an addiction without side effects or collateral damage.

PHYSICAL PROBLEMS—Smoking causes cancer, heart disease, stroke, lung diseases, diabetes, and chronic obstructive pulmonary disease (COPD), which includes emphysema and chronic bronchitis. Smoking also increases the risk of contracting tuberculosis, certain eye diseases, and problems of the immune system, including rheumatoid arthritis. It interferes with the senses of taste and smell. Attempts to quit can instigate a withdrawal component that places a tremendous strain on the body's organs, the muscles, and the neurological system. Withdrawal from nicotine occurs after every cigarette smoked.

MENTAL ISSUES—Nicotine use is associated with higher levels of conditions like ADHD. Vaping can worsen symptoms of depression.

SOCIAL PROBLEMS—While those who smoke and vape tend to interact with each other on a social level while partaking in their addiction, interactions with non-smokers, those who don't smoke or vape decrease since those people usually don't want to be around the smoke or vapors. Some people express their disdain for those who are addicted to nicotine and may choose not to socialize with them.

LEGAL PROBLEMS—For the most part, there are no legal concerns with smoking and vaping. Legal issues may occur if cigarettes are purchased in a tax-free state with the intent to resell them or in quantities over the accepted limit for that state. There can be legal trouble if a nicotine addict steals cigarettes or vape products or the money to purchase them.

FINANCIAL CONCERNS—A smoker who smokes a pack of cigarettes per day may spend close to $3,000 a year on their nicotine habit. Other nicotine-delivery systems may be less expensive but still take a significant chunk out of one's spending money.

FAMILY AND RELATIONSHIP ISSUES—There are no significant issues related to family concerns and relationships. Considering the amount of money spent on the addiction and whether or not other family members are also smokers, there can be a strain on relationships that are financially based. Also, nonsmokers tend to resent the debris left behind by smokers and the foul odors that can linger. It is important to note that, like any other addiction, addicts can be selfish and lack consideration of other people's feelings about their nicotine addiction. This can lead to arguments and resentment from family and friends.

EMPLOYMENT PROBLEMS—There seem to be no problems with employment and smoking. Though most businesses have a no-smoking policy in the place of business, it is not uncommon for companies to designate areas for smokers to use on breaks.

CHANGES IN SOCIAL LIFE—With so many nonsmokers in social settings, smokers these days are usually expected to leave the social interaction and step outside to smoke. This may result in their missing key events, such as being outside while everyone is singing "Happy Birthday" or getting up from the dinner table for a smoke between courses. Depending on the people involved, nonsmokers may have problems with the smoker smelling like smoke when they return to the social setting.

LYING—Lying is also not seen as a significant factor in nicotine use. It is not uncommon for smokers to underreport the number of cigarettes they smoke and the money they are spending on their addiction.

ACCOUNTABILITY ISSUES—If someone has a significant nicotine addiction, they may rush through a task or take longer to complete it because they are taking time away from the task to smoke or vape.

PERSONALITY CHANGES—One study found that individuals who smoked users were more likely to exhibit an increase in neuroticism. Smokers also displayed declines in extroversion, openness, agreeableness, and conscientiousness. See https://neurosciencenews.com/smoking-personality-changes-14383/

ANGER AND VIOLENCE—Withdrawal from nicotine creates irritability and quick, impulsive reactions. These could be precursors to anger and violence.

Everyone experiences addiction according to their unique set of circumstances. Sporadic users of nicotine, such as weekend smokers or those who smoke or vape just a few times a day, experience less significant problems than those who smoke more often. Also, those who smoke and vape infrequently do not experience withdrawal symptoms with the same intensity as heavy users. Heavier smokers and vapers will experience swings in moods and tolerance levels in the interval between uses. The critical takeaway is that regardless of how much you smoke or how you do it, nicotine addiction is real; it is not without severe drawbacks and health risks, and it can have a profound impact on the way you live your life.

COLLATERAL DAMAGE

For quite a long time, no one paid much attention to how much damage cigarettes we're causing. Throughout most of the twentieth century, smoking was allowed in public places, and outside of the potential cancer risk, little was spoken about in terms of personal and public health. In the late 1990s and early 2000s, some states implemented comprehensive smoking bans that prohibited smoking in most workplaces and all public places, including previously exempted bars and restaurants. Today, very few public establishments allow smoking in public areas. Some set aside areas where people may smoke without affecting the clean air of those close to them.

Sooner or later, every smoker or vaper is going to experience the physical damage that smoking and vaping can cause. It will produce limitations in physical exertion and may be costly on a financial level. For example, if a person smoked or vaped every day for more than twenty years, it would be nearly equivalent to an American worker's current average annual salary. These are not costs the nicotine addicts incur alone if they have a family to support or contribute to.

Smokers and vapers aren't always considerate regarding where they indulge in their habit. Many will argue that they have the right to smoke or vape in their own home, in their car, or outdoor areas, stating that if someone doesn't like it, they can go somewhere else. This can impact the social relationships between users and non-users. Moreover, if someone cannot leave the proximity (such as a child who lives in the home or rides in the car), they can be exposed to secondhand smoke and vapor.

Withdrawal from nicotine is well documented, and most of the focus on quitting smoking or vaping is on the withdrawal that takes place when the addict attempts to stop using. However, as I mentioned earlier, smoking and vaping cause "mini withdrawals" that occur between each smoking or vaping episode. Smokers will often say that smoking them "calms them down." For someone who is addicted to nicotine, in the twenty or thirty minutes after they smoke or vape, their body goes into withdrawal and begins to crave the drug once again. If they indulge in that craving, the withdrawal symptoms are eased, making it seem as if the smoking relaxes them.

Without nicotine, the addict becomes irritable, demanding, temperamental, and physically challenged. Family and friends will be on the receiving end of the addict's ill temper, and once again, the consequences stretch beyond the addict to affect other people. Worse yet, if the nicotine addict is also addicted to caffeine, alcohol, or both, and those other drugs are not close by, the situation can get volatile, and everyone around the addict, who may or may not realize this is occurring, is negatively affected.

Some smokers and vapors are considerate enough to keep their addiction away from those close to them. They will keep things clean, not subject others to secondhand smoke or vapor, and even make sure that it doesn't affect the family's finances, using only their personal spending money to support their habit. Other people are not so fortunate. The nicotine addicts in their lives have no concern about such things, and they must experience the inconsiderate behavior of these addicts daily.

Even if these more significant forms of collateral damage are minimized, there is still the stench that remains from tobacco use and the cigarette butts, vape cartridges, and other paraphernalia that are part of the smoking and vaping experiences. Once again, those around you who are not addicted to nicotine experience whatever you choose to leave behind.

SUMMING IT UP

For decades, the tobacco industry was successful in convincing people that there was no such thing as nicotine addiction. The word "nicotine" was rarely mentioned. It was fashionable to smoke, and there was little attention paid to the downside of smoking.

Quitting nicotine is one of the most challenging drugs to quit. It can cause a tremendous amount of damage physically, financially, and to varying extents to those people close to the addict. It is essential to look at smoking and vaping as the powerful nicotine addictions they are and the effects they are having throughout one's life. Honesty is imperative. It's time to stop minimizing the effects of nicotine addiction. Ask yourself these questions:

➤ How is nicotine affecting my health?

➤ How much money am I spending on nicotine products every week? Multiply that by fifty-two to see your annual spending rate, then by how many years you have used those products.

➤ Ask yourself if you are a considerate user. Do you make sure no one is near you when you smoke or vape? Also, do you ensure that the area you smoke or vape in will not be quickly occupied by others who may be affected by or offended by the smell?

➤ Are there times when you could be doing other, more productive things and must remove yourself from them so you can satisfy your addiction?

➤ Do you get up in the middle of the night to have a cigarette or vape?

➤ Is the first thing you do in the morning and the last thing you do at night smoke or vape?

➤ Are other people complaining about your smoking or vaping and giving you intelligent reasons regarding how it is affecting you and them?

➤ Are you defensive about your nicotine addiction and refuse to listen to other's good advice?

➤ Has a doctor or other medical professional told you that smoking or vaping is affecting your health, but you are not to follow their advice?

➤ Are you unwilling to look at any information about the health risks, other dangers, and collateral damage associated with your nicotine addiction?

Examining any addiction demands honesty and a willingness to look at information that may suggest that you stop what you are doing. Regardless of what you may have learned about nicotine addiction, nicotine is still a drug; it is highly addictive and can have disastrous effects on your health and what occurs in your family. Some drugs are prescribed to treat serious ailments and must be taken. Even those drugs have side effects. However, at least when a drug is taken for health reasons, it treats a problem. Nicotine is *not* one of those drugs.

"According to the National Institute on Drug Abuse (NIDA), nicotine creates a temporary feeling of well-being and relaxation and increases heart rate and the amount of oxygen the heart uses. As nicotine enters the body, it causes a surge of endorphins, which are chemicals that help to relieve stress and pain and improve mood. The euphoria, however, is mild and short lasting. Ultimately, the adverse effects on one's health far outweigh the short-term euphoric advantages.

If you are thinking about quitting smoking and would like help, call 1 (800) 784-8669. Everything is confidential.

 ## TIME TO TAKE ACTION

1. Review the list of questions presented in the previous section. Be honest about whether they apply to you.

2. Keep track of how much money you spend on nicotine-related products in one week. Multiply that number by fifty-two to give you your yearly nicotine use financial estimate.

3. Ask the people close to you if you're smoking or vaping is a problem for them. If they answer yes, ask them how it affects them and begin considering that.

4. Make an appointment with your primary care physician to determine if smoking or vaping has impacted your health.

5. If you decide to stop smoking or vaping, do it under the guidance of your physician or therapist. Reducing the amount you use each day in small increments is a good idea. Smoking-reduction programs, hypnosis, and acupuncture can also help you stop.

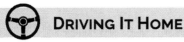 **DRIVING IT HOME**

Smoking's harmful effects went unaddressed for decades because it was so accepted on the world stage for centuries before its harmful effects were known. While vaping's popularity is increasing, just like cigarettes, it can have a severe impact on your health due to the toxic and carcinogenic ingredients contained in the vaping liquid. With the research available to understand what nicotine addiction does to the human body and the collateral damage it can cause to family and friends, try to look at it as a viable addiction as well as one of the most challenging addictions to quit. Treat nicotine use as the addiction it is, and do your best to remove yourself from its clutches. Life is too short to let an empty addiction tear it apart.

YOUR DECLARATION IS: *I will treat nicotine use as the addiction it is, and I will remove it from my life!*

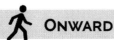 **ONWARD**

Prescription drug use has grown to epidemic proportions throughout the world. In the next chapter, I will examine prescription drugs and how damage can be minimized when they are used appropriately. I will also look at what happens when they are abused and how the abuse can lead to a severe life-threatening addiction.

◇◇◇◇◇◇◇◇◇◇◇◇

CHAPTER 5

Prescription Drugs— Savior and Grim Reaper

They are the consummate good, bad, and ugly. They can cure what ails you, steal your identity, and turn your world into a living hell.

PROCESSES TO EMPLOY: Brutal Honesty, I Over E, Present-Understand-Fix, Slowing Down Life's Pace, Internal Focus, Fact-Finding, Honesty, Patience, Truth-Telling, Belief, Listening, Trust

---

SINCE 2000, THE USE OF PRESCRIPTION DRUGS around the world has skyrocketed. In the late 1980s, approximately 5 percent of the people I counseled were all on medications for anxiety and depression. Today, that number has ballooned to over 70 percent. Drug companies are pushing these medications at a pace we have never seen before. Commercial advertising spots occur regularly, promising increased health by taking those medications. Even though side effects are stated at the end of the commercial spot, people don't seem to care. A quick fix is a quick fix; many people want what they want when they want it, and their need for immediate gratification opens the door for the empty pharmaceutical company promises.

The movement away from sustained therapeutic approaches without medications continues, and all too often, people are seeking out physicians who are willing to quickly prescribe medications before their patients have had the opportunity to address the causes of the problem with counseling professionals. The increase in prescription drug usage is alarming, and if big pharma has its way, the trend will continue.

Prescription Drug Abuse

The use of prescription drugs has its advantages but also some serious disadvantages. Prescriptions are designed to help treat physical ailments, but their side effects can be disastrous. [4]

> Among Americans aged twelve years and older, 37.309 million were current illegal drug users (used within the last thirty days).

> 13.5% of Americans aged twelve and overused drugs in the last month, a 3.8% increase year-over-year.

> 59.277 million, or 21.4% of people aged twelve and over, have used illegal drugs or misused prescription drugs within the last year.

> 138.543 million or 50% of people aged twelve and over have illicitly used drugs in their lifetime.

> 25.4% of illegal drug users have a drug disorder.

> 24.7% of those with drug disorders have an opioid disorder; this includes prescription pain relievers or "pain killers" and heroin

> 6% of Americans over age 12 abuse prescription drugs in a year.

> Four out of five pharmacy-filled prescriptions are opioids.

> 12% of prescription drug abusers are addicted.

> The following table illustrates the number of annual prescription drug abusers. The table provides the various prescription drugs, the annual number of abusers worldwide, the number of abusers who obtained prescriptions for the drugs, and the percentage of Americans abusing the medications.

The most concerning increases in prescription drug usage occurred in the early 2000s when the opiate epidemic took thousands of lives and led U.S. states and the federal government to sanction physicians who were either overprescribing these medications or prescribing them when they were not needed. Today, though it is more difficult to obtain these medications, they are always available on the black market.

TABLE 5.1. PRESCRIPTION DRUG USE PERCENTAGES

Drug Type	Annual Abusers	% Among Rx Abusers	% Among Americans*
Painkillers	9.7 million	59.5%	3.43%
Opioids	9.3 million	57.1%	3.29%
Sedatives	5.9 million	36.2%	2.08%
Stimulants	4.9 million	30.1%	0.73%
Benzodiazepines	4.8 million	29.4%	1.70%
All Prescription Drugs	16.3 million		

As noted earlier, the primary drugs of abuse are painkillers, opioids, sedatives, stimulants, and benzodiazepines. The drugs all have one common attribute: They help their users feel better quickly. Unfortunately, they are also highly addictive, and addiction to these medications occurs quicker than any other legal drug. In this chapter, I will focus on prescription medications that can lead to addiction. In Chapter 6, I will cover two other opiates responsible for thousands of lost lives—heroin and fentanyl.

THE PROGRESSION

1. A person is introduced to the drug for the first time. This could be at a party, by a friend or family member, or by taking someone's medication when they are unaware that this is happening. It could also be prescribed medication by one's primary care physician or surgeon.

2. The person either experiments with the drug provided or takes it as directed by their doctor.

3. The drug, being used medicinally to address chronic pain, anxiety, temporary pain after surgery or a medical procedure, or recreationally, begins to produce a state of euphoria.

4. Feeling the euphoric effects of the drug, the person may request additional prescriptions, saying that the pain or other symptoms have not subsided. If used recreationally, the source is contacted to obtain more.

5. Whether used medicinally or recreationally, the person's body and mind are now adjusting to the physical and euphoric effects of the drug.

6. The user is beginning to believe they need the medication either because their symptoms are still present or because their life is not as enjoyable without the drug.

7. Other people tell the user they may be dependent, but denial causes them to believe otherwise.

8. The user begins to feel withdrawal effects when the drug runs out, though the effects at this point are not serious.

9. The user continues to use, and now the amount of the drug used is beginning to increase. Dependence is becoming observable.

10. As the tolerance for the drug develops, the user, now becoming addicted, needs to use more of the drug and more often to get the same effects.

11. The withdrawal between uses is becoming more serious as physical tremors, intense irritability, sweats, body aches, difficulty consuming food, and sleepless nights have begun.

12. Now realizing the dependence on the drug, the addict rationalizes the need for the drug and continues to do what they can to obtain it.

13. Some addicts will "doctor shop" to obtain prescriptions from doctors who are not aware of their dependence on the drug.

14. As the supply becomes more difficult to obtain, the addict begins to take risks such as using other people's prescriptions, stealing from others and businesses, embezzling, stealing from family and friends, robbery, forging prescriptions, and anything necessary to acquire the drug.

15. In more severe cases, the addict may be hospitalized or incarcerated, and in some cases, an overdose of the drug results in death.

People who never had a problem with medications can quickly become addicted to prescription medications. They could be the opiates and painkillers that are prescribed after a tooth is extracted or a minor surgery. Often, medications are prescribed for short periods after these events. However, for major surgeries, the length of the prescription could be significantly longer.

Physicians and surgeons do try to avoid prescribing stronger opioids like hydrocodone, oxycodone, and Percocet (oxycodone). They may attempt to treat pain with larger doses of acetaminophen (e.g., Tylenol) with codeine for a short period, for example. However, codeine is also addictive, so it is crucial to monitor the length of time this drug is used. Amphetamines are often prescribed for weight loss, ADD and ADHD, and narcolepsy (a sleep disorder). Once again, the danger of prescribing too much of the medication over a longer period can be dangerous. Many amphetamine-based drugs are being prescribed by psychiatrists who tend to have more knowledge and experience regarding their usage, but this does not mean the patient will not become dependent.

Overuse and addiction to prescription medications are a clear indicator of how insidious and powerful addiction is. Becoming addicted to prescription medications can affect the strongest of minds and people who rarely, if ever, put any substance in their bodies. Addiction to these medications can sneak up on you since, many times, they are prescribed by a qualified professional to treat a medical condition. The time it takes to become addicted could be as little as a week or ten days. Be very careful with prescription drugs.

IN THE CLUTCHES

No addiction is free from the problems and side effects that develop from continued use. What follows is a list of the effects that one can experience from addiction to any drug or activity. Different addictions can lead to different problems as you will see as we continue.

PHYSICAL PROBLEMS—All drugs have side effects. In addition to their addictive components, painkillers, opioids, sedatives, stimulants, and benzodiazepines all affect the brain. All except stimulants slow brain processes, and over time, they can all do irreparable damage. Stimulants increase neurological functioning, but they also put a tremendous strain on the brain and the nervous system. Stimulants can cause paranoia and perceptual difficulties, while all of these medications alter the way the brain perceives and organizes information. Throughout the body, there are effects on the heart and cardiovascular system, the muscles, the skeletal system, and even the excretory system, especially with opioid use. These medications interfere with sleep habits with some having a negative impact on one's nutrition, and all impact the liver and kidneys, the purifying organs in the body.

MENTAL HEALTH ISSUES—Chronic use of these medications can lead to anxiety and depression, especially painkillers, opioids, and sedatives. Even in the case of benzodiazepines, which can be prescribed to treat conditions like anxiety, it is not uncommon for the dosage to be increased as one becomes more tolerant of the drug, leading to enhanced side effects such as memory issues, difficulty focusing, and difficulty organizing information. As the addiction progresses, personal hygiene can be compromised, as the addicts lose the focus they need to care for their bodies.

COMMUNICATION PROBLEMS—As the dose of the medication increases and addiction begins to set in, communication suffers as people withdraw, isolate, or, in some cases, become more argumentative. Also, with the perceptual and organizational difficulties affecting information processing, communication is often inefficient, fragmented, and abusive.

LEGAL PROBLEMS—As use progresses to abuse and finally to addiction, and addicts are unable to secure prescriptions, they may turn to alternate sources to obtain the drug, usually drug dealers. Legal problems typically include possession of controlled substances, assaults, theft and receiving stolen property, shoplifting, and, at times, home invasions.

FINANCIAL CONCERNS—While the prescriptions are still in force, medical benefits may offset the price of the drugs. However, when prescriptions cannot be secured, these drugs are purchased through friends and dealers. It's not uncommon for a prescription drug addict to spend between $500 and $1,000 per week to support their habit. As the addiction progresses, household bills are not paid, precious items are sold, and, for some, bankruptcy may result.

FAMILY AND RELATIONSHIP ISSUES—Addiction puts tremendous stress on the addict and their family members. Addicts can become angry, verbally or physically abusive, steal from family members, are not always accountable concerning finances and household responsibilities, and, at times, require hospitalizations and inpatient programs to address the problem. Communication suffers, and there is distance that grows between the addict and family members.

EMPLOYMENT PROBLEMS—When the abuse progresses to the point of addiction, addicts keep very poor living schedules. Memory and accountability suffer. They are often late to work, may leave early or call out sick, have poor work habits, and have difficult relationships with other employees. Prescription drug addicts often lose their jobs and may skip from job to job as employability is reduced.

CHANGES IN SOCIAL LIFE—When prescription drug abuse becomes an addiction, people tend to remove themselves from positive social situations. This may occur with family and close friends. They may isolate, spend time with other people who are addicted, and do whatever they can to avoid situations where they must spend time with others who are not abusing drugs.

LYING—As with all addictions, lying about the continued use of the drug, how much of the drug is being taken, how often it is being taken, financial matters, stealing from family members, and anything that helps support the addiction becomes a standard way to live. Addicts are secretive and will keep others as far from the truth as they can.

ACCOUNTABILITY ISSUES—Addicts are anything but accountable. The longer they are addicted, the less they are thinking about what they need to be doing. They will procrastinate and do anything in their power to avoid being accountable since the responsibilities that come with accountability will interfere with their drug use and the euphoria that is so important to them. Also, with their physical abilities being compromised, they can have difficulties performing the responsibilities associated with accountability.

PERSONALITY CHANGES—Anytime a person is dependent on a prescription drug and must do what they need to do to obtain their drug of choice, their personality will change. They will experience periods of euphoria followed by periods of withdrawal. They will have mood swings, difficulty sleeping, and are often irritable and intolerant. They are resistant to advice and blame others for their difficulties. They may experience periods of depression followed by periods of anxiety and are reactive in even the simplest of circumstances.

ANGER AND VIOLENCE—When an addict is in withdrawal or obsessed with obtaining the drugs they need for that particular day, any interference can bring on anger and the potential for violence. Also, withdrawal instigates pain, and pain is a natural precursor for severe mood changes. Even when they are not in withdrawal, their fluctuating moods are a breeding ground for anger and violence.

COLLATERAL DAMAGE

No one escapes the damage that is part of prescription drug addiction. For some prescription drug addicts, obsessive-compulsive behavior has always been a problem. It may have manifested in other addictions such as shopping, work, food, or other obsessive endeavors. For them, the move to prescription drug addiction can be a natural progression. Two types of people become addicted to prescription drugs:

1. People who have had issues with other substances or other addictions.

2. People who never seemed to have had a problem with any other substance or addiction.

Some addicts who use street drugs may turn to prescription medications because they are legal and a prescription is available for them. In some cases, physicians might have been aware of a past problem but underestimated the potential for an addictive response. In other cases, a prescription medication was prescribed to address a problem, with no indication that there would be an issue. Unfortunately, after taking the medication for a few weeks, a dependence developed.

Regardless of how an addiction begins, the addict will experience most of the addiction-related problems mentioned earlier. Also, family and others close to them will be affected by their addiction. Those affected include parents, significant others, children, close relatives, friends, employers and other employees, and business partners. On various levels, these people will experience communication problems, problems with accountability, lying, stealing, absenteeism, binges, verbal and or physical violence, financial issues, and personality changes.

In the cases of someone who has been addicted for a long time, the change to a prescription medication means that family members will experience a continuation of what has been a way of life for some time. For other people who have been prescribed the drug and then became addicted shortly after that, this may all be new to them. This person who was responsible, respectful, engaged, and someone you could depend on suddenly became someone who spent the family finances, was angry and aggressive, displayed personality changes, stole from them, and lied about everything.

Family members who are involved with a person who is addicted to prescription medications can find themselves carrying the brunt of the family responsibilities and being on the receiving end of negative and often hostile behaviors. Employers may experience work reduction issues, absenteeism, and having to remove the person from their employment. Bill collectors may call the house. Friends will experience distance that they never experienced before.

There may be hospital and rehabilitation visits, individual and family counseling, involvement with the law with court dates, probation, and incarceration. In the more severe cases, families will lose homes or, at the very least, in some cases, declare bankruptcy to keep ownership of their homes. The worst-case scenario occurs when the addict loses their life to the addiction. The emotional toll addiction takes on family and others involved in the prescription drug addict's life can be horrible. It is not uncommon for them to require the services of a counselor or a 12-step program to help them through the damage the addiction caused.

SUMMING IT UP

Though many prescription drug addicts may be innocent regarding their use of the medication and become addicted after a few weeks of use, it doesn't change the collateral damage. The advice here is simple: If you have addiction issues, make sure your physician understands this and that you are consistently monitored while using the medication. The potential for addiction to them can be extremely high.

If you are prescribed any of the medications mentioned in this chapter for a medical condition, stop using the medication when your prescription runs out. If you are having issues, it is essential to report this to your physician quickly so help may be provided if you need a step-down program to stop using the drug. Prescription drug addiction kills thousands of people each year. It doesn't have to include you. If you think you are dependent on a prescription medication, let your physician know immediately.

For substance abuse treatment information, contact the Substance Abuse and Mental Health Services Administration's (SAMHSA) National Helpline at 1-800-662-HELP (4357). Everything is confidential.

 TIME TO TAKE ACTION

1. Before you obtain a prescription for any of the drugs discussed in this chapter, make sure your physician can review your family history to determine if there may be addiction-related problems.

2. Take your prescription medication only as long as it was initially prescribed.

3. If you are having problems with withdrawal from a drug, consult your physician immediately.

4. If a family member or someone close to you is having difficulty withdrawing from a prescribed medication, help them obtain medical help immediately.

5. If you are on a prescribed medication and know that you are addicted to it, consult your physician or go to an emergency room immediately.

6. Avoid purchasing any prescribed medications from street-level dealers. Their product may be laced with additives and other drugs you are not aware of.

7. Take note of the progression from initial use to dependence presented earlier in this chapter. If you think you are progressing from use to addiction, either get help or have someone help you to do so. Start with your family physician.

8. If you notice behavioral changes, items or money missing from your home, bills not being paid, or any changes noted earlier, it may be a sign that someone in your home is addicted. Open a discussion with everyone in your home to determine if addiction is the problem.

9. Talk about the problem. Addiction counselors can help, and so can support people like Narcotics Anonymous. Al-Anon meetings are good for family members, or you can use the national abuse hotline.

10. Never let a prescription drug addiction go untreated. If you see it, it is better to err on the side of caution and get help. You can start with their family physician, call the SAMHSA hotline (800-662-HELP [4357]), or, in more severe cases, go to an emergency room.

DRIVING IT HOME

Prescription drugs are designed to treat physical and, at times, emotional problems. They were never meant to be used recreationally. In many cases, it does not take much to become addicted, and the addiction to these drugs can be severe and horrifying. If you are abusing prescription medications, it is essential to get help quickly. If you know someone who is abusing prescription medications or you feel may be addicted, approach them and discuss the matter with them. Just because these drugs are manufactured to address medical problems and are prescribed by a physician does not mean they don't carry a serious potential for addiction. If you are unsure how to help yourself or someone else, call the SAMHSA hotline (800-662-HELP [4357]). The faster you get help, the better the chance for recovery.

YOUR DECLARATION IS: *I will be careful about taking prescription drugs. If I need help stopping, I will get it immediately!*

 ONWARD

In the next chapter, I will take a close look at heroin and fentanyl addiction. I will discuss the personality change that occurs as addiction commences, the damage to the body, and its long-term effects on the life of the user and those close to them.

◇◇◇◇◇◇◇◇◇◇◇◇

CHAPTER 6

Heroin and Fentanyl— The (Not So) Peaceful Route to Death

It is the perfect marriage between Nirvana and the devil.
In the end, the devil wins.

PROCESSES TO EMPLOY: Brutal Honesty, I Over E, Present-Understand-Fix, Slowing Down Life's Pace, Internal Focus, Fact-Finding, Honesty, Patience, Truth-Telling, Belief, Listening, Trust

---

➤ Heroin is a potent analgesic, five to ten times more potent than morphine. It is one of the most widely used street drugs. When one thinks of heroin, the brain usually conjures up visions of addicts injecting their arms and other body parts with syringes. However, this opiate derivative can also be snorted and smoked. It provides a highly euphoric state while rendering its user unable to perform even the simplest tasks.

➤ Opiates are chemical compounds extracted or refined from natural plant matter. Other examples of opiates include opium, morphine, and codeine. Heroin is a morphinan opioid substance synthesized from the dried latex of the Papaver somniferum plant; it is mainly used as a recreational drug for its euphoric effects. Approximately 12 percent of opium is made up of the analgesic alkaloid morphine, which is processed chemically to produce heroin and other synthetic opioids for medicinal use and the illegal drug trade.

Fentanyl is an extremely potent synthetic opioid that was first developed in the 1960s. Being a strong painkiller, fentanyl is used medically for breakthrough pain that doesn't respond to conventional painkillers. It is also used to treat severe chronic pain. Fentanyl works by mimicking the body's natural endorphins, hormones that block pain receptors in the brain. Fentanyl is fifty times more potent than heroin and a hundred times stronger than morphine. It is often added to heroin to boost its potency. Also, it is considerably cheaper than heroin, so those dealing the drug often add it to heroin to beef up their product without informing the user.

THE STATISTICS

Here are recent statistics regarding heroin:[5]

➤ Deaths due to heroin overdoses have significantly increased since 2010. From 2012 to 2014, the rate of heroin overdose deaths nearly doubled. After 2014, the death rate remained in the tens of thousands.

➤ Over 14,000 Americans die annually from overdosing on heroin. Over 8,700 people die annually from overdosing on heroin and synthetic opioids other than methadone, and over 5,200 people die annually from overdosing on heroin without taking synthetic opioids other than methadone.

➤ From 2021 to 2022, the heroin overdose death rate decreased nearly 36%

➤ 1.7 million deaths occur annually from overdoses of heroin without taking synthetic opioids other than methadone.

➤ Fentanyl is increasingly responsible for the growing number of accidental overdoses. Currently, more than 67% of drug overdoses involve fentanyl.

➤ Almost three deaths occur annually from overdoses on heroin and synthetic opioids other than methadone for every 100,000 people.

THE PROGRESSION

1. The person, usually a casual substance user, is asked if they want to try heroin, and for a while, they refuse.

2. The person snorts heroin for the first time. This usually occurs with friends and acquaintances who already use the drug.

3. The person likes the effects of the drug and uses it for a second time, usually with the same people.

4. The drug is snorted over a short period, producing the same euphoric results.

5. After some coercing, the new user smokes heroin for the first time. The euphoria is enhanced, and the person continues smoking the drug.

6. Other heroin addicts who inject the drug ask the user if they'd like to try to "shoot up."

7. Initially, the user rejects the idea, feeling as though they will not be a heroin addict if they don't shoot up.

8. The user continues to snort and smoke the drug, but not every day.

9. The user begins to use the drug more often and starts wondering what the effects would be if they injected it just once.

10. Someone tells them that they will shoot them up for the first time, using a small amount of the drug. Finally, the user agrees.

11. The euphoric rush experienced during the first intravenous use produces a quick and potent state of euphoria; the person understands the rush.

12. Heroin is injected a second time, again, by someone else.

13. The user starts intravenous use, now injecting themselves.

14. The addiction is in full swing as the addictive cycle begins.

15. The addict now wants to get high as often as possible. The addiction has progressed to the point that withdrawal has become painful and, at times, prolonged.

16. Not having the funds to continue with the addiction, the addict begins to search for alternate methods to secure the drug. Withdrawal events begin.

17. 17. Withdrawal symptoms from the heroine include sweats, tremors, vomiting, head and body aches, and fever. The addict will do anything now to avoid withdrawal and "get right."

18. The addict will use as much as they can, as often as they can, at the cost of everything else in their life.

Not everyone goes through the same progression. For some people who may have experienced more prolonged or higher dose exposure to addictive drugs, such as prescription drugs, especially those that produce opiate-like euphoria, the progression might be quicker. Many people use drugs for recreational purposes, and some may use heroin sporadically because they want an occasional euphoric experience but are trying to be careful about not becoming addicted to the drug.

Fentanyl, which is so much more powerful than heroin, has a much faster progression. Since it is so potent, addiction can occur quickly. Overdoses occur because the human body can only take small amounts of fentanyl, and it should always be administered under the care of a medical professional. Because fentanyl is often added to heroin, heroin users are more at risk for a fentanyl overdose.

IN THE CLUTCHES

No addiction is free from the problems and side effects that develop from continued use. What follows is a list of the effects that one can experience from addiction to any drug or activity. Different addictions can lead to different problems, as you will see as we continue.

PHYSICAL PROBLEMS—These issues can include liver disease, pulmonary infections, arthritis/rheumatological problems, collapsed veins, chronic constipation, depression, kidney disease, infection of heart valves and lining, skin abscesses or infections, increased risk of contracting hepatitis and HIV as well as other bloodborne viruses.

MENTAL HEALTH ISSUES—These issues can include severe depression, a sense of hopelessness that nothing will change, feelings of emptiness and despair, inability to sleep, anxiety and panic with feelings of dread, emotional fatigue, and suicidal ideation.

COMMUNICATION PROBLEMS—Addicts tend to be poor communicators. When they are under the influence of the drug, the depressant effects on the brain make communication almost impossible. When they are not using the drug and in withdrawal, they are often angry and in pain, and their communication style is agitated, fragmented, and verbally abusive.

LEGAL PROBLEMS—Heroin addicts often find themselves in difficult circumstances with legal authorities. Charges include possession, possession with intent to deliver, burglary, theft and receiving stolen property, assaults (during withdrawal), prostitution, forgery, and vagrancy.

FINANCIAL CONCERNS—Heroin addiction is very expensive, and only those who are wealthy can tolerate its financial drain. The average heroin addict spends between $80 and $200 per day. They will do without basic necessities, often unable to buy the food they need to survive. Heroin addicts are often in financial distress and often rely on others to pay for or supply even their most rudimentary necessities.

FAMILY AND RELATIONSHIP ISSUES—Heroin addiction creates a tremendous amount of stress and anxiety. Family members experience the addict's severe mood swings and communication issues while grappling with their financial concerns, legal problems, overdoses, and hospitalizations. At times, the addict's family may find their safety compromised. Family members often need to practice tough love and remove the addict from their household. The loss of the addict to a heroin overdose is devastating and initiates a grieving process that can last for years.

EMPLOYMENT PROBLEMS—Because they are typically high or in withdrawal, heroin addicts have difficulty maintaining employment. They usually cannot adhere to work schedules and are rarely efficient when they do show up to work. They are generally terminated and remain unemployed for long periods since they do not interview well, even if they are looking for a job.

CHANGES IN SOCIAL LIFE—The heroin addict's social life revolves around the drug. They maintain few, if any, positive relationships, and most of their acquaintances are also drug addicts and/or dealers. From their point of view, there is no point in spending time with anyone who cannot help them get high.

LYING—Lying is the hallmark of an addict's way of life. They lie not only about their addiction but about anything that may hold them accountable or interfere with their addiction. Often, their lies are elaborate and quite believable to others who do not understand the dynamics of addiction.

ACCOUNTABILITY ISSUES—There is almost no accountability with the heroin addict. Once the addiction takes hold, they do not possess the cognitive or physical ability to carry through on any issues that call for them to be accountable and responsible.

PERSONALITY CHANGES—Heroin addiction instigates a severe personality change, including frequent impulsivity and recklessness, self-doubt, manipulation, laziness, arrogance, disrespect, disorganization, impatience, distrustfulness, irresponsibility, and criticalness.

ANGER AND VIOLENCE—While under the influence of heroin, it isn't the norm for the addict to be angry and violent. Conversely, when they are in withdrawal and pain, they will quickly become angry and resort to any method, including violence, to obtain the drug.

COLLATERAL DAMAGE

Heroin addiction can take family members on a terrifying, never-ending emotional roller-coaster ride. They may exhaust every possible resource to save their loved one, often unsuccessfully. (It is difficult to save someone who doesn't want to be saved.) They will often clean up after the addict during withdrawal, pay fines and court costs, bail them out of jail, and almost go broke in the process. They will often lose sleep to respond to a call in the middle of the night to rescue the addict. They will appear at court hearings and do their best to keep them out of jail, even when they know they did something wrong. They will do their best to get them healthy and then watch them squander every effort as they return to their heroin-induced euphoric mirage.

Emotionally, family members become exhausted and devastated. They do not realize how far down the addiction pulls them in. Before they know it, they are defending the addict's irresponsible behavior. They explain away their manipulations. They will lie for them and lose sleep worrying about them. In the end, they will feel as though they were sucked so deep into the addiction that they were defending the very way of life that was killing their loved one.

Intellectually, they will make decisions they never thought they would make. They will do what they should never do as they try to save their addicted family member. They will begin to experience difficulties focusing and separating fact from fiction. They will feel victimized, and their powers of rational thought will be ripped from them. They, themselves, will begin to discount the factual information presented by other family members and friends and by addiction professionals. They will find themselves in denial, rationalizing the behavior of the addict. Ultimately, they will feel betrayed, used, ashamed, and embarrassed.

The best-case scenario is that they will go through all of this, and somewhere down the line, the addict will get help and enter into recovery. Manipulated and used, the family members can at least wrap their arms around their addicted loved one and hope that recovery is something they embrace. They live waiting for the phone to ring, and in the worst-case scenario, all their efforts will be for naught, and they will lose their loved one. When that happens, they often lose themselves.

SUMMING IT UP

The fight against heroin addiction is one of the most difficult wars to win. It is a fight against a relentless enemy that eventually controls its victims' bodies, minds, and emotions. Reduced to mere shells of their prior self, the addict is crushed by an addiction that takes no prisoners. Lost and directionless, the addict's loved ones are caught in a world of darkness and potential doom.

There is help available, and if there is any chance to save the heroin addict, it will be by using a network of people who know what they are doing. Counselors with mental health and strong addiction knowledge and treatment skills are essential. Narcotics Anonymous and the support an addict can receive from recovering addicts can provide a life-saving program that will always be there for them. Counseling for family members is also essential to help them understand the dynamics of the addiction, make the early decisions that could save their family member's life, and keep them from losing theirs. Al-Anon is a good support for family members.

If someone in your family is addicted to heroin, call the National Drug Helpline at (844) 289-0879. It is free and confidential.

 TIME TO TAKE ACTION

1. If you are addicted to heroin, or if it is a problem in your life, don't waste time getting help. You can refer to the list in In The Clutches section to assess the problems heroin or fentanyl are causing in your life. If you don't know an addiction specialist, you can start with your primary-care physician, go to the closest emergency room, and you can also call the national drug helpline listed above.

2. Never keep your or someone else's addiction a secret. Too many people lose the fight with heroin addiction because they waited too long to get help. If the signs are there, or any changes make you suspicious, make the initial calls for help.

3. If your family member is fighting a heroin addiction, they need help, but so do you. Family members rarely, if ever, can handle this alone. Your ability to help your loved one is only as strong as your ability to help yourself. Share your information with physicians, addiction specialists, or support people. Let them help you.

4. Take time to acquire as much information as you can about heroin addiction and treatment options. Get your information from reliable addiction professionals and treatment programs.

5. Familiarize yourself with the treatment resources in your area. This should also include contact information for any drug-treatment programs in your area or the closest ones to you, as well as contact information for the Narcotics Anonymous chapters nearby. Also, write down all emergency numbers, including those for the police department, the hospital, ambulance services, and advocates who can help you and your family. Don't wait until the point of crisis; have these numbers handy in case that time arrives.

6. Don't try to diagnose if someone has a drug problem. Look for changes in their behavior like isolation, hygiene changes, communication difficulties, anger and violence, health issues, and anything different from their typical baseline behaviors. If these changes are occurring, contact your primary-care physician or an addiction specialist and talk about your observations with them.

7. Talk about the problem. Addiction counselors can help, and so can support people like Narcotics Anonymous. Al-Anon meetings are good for family members, or you can use the national abuse hotline.

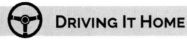

DRIVING IT HOME

Heroin addiction is one of the most devastating problems families can deal with. It is so important to move away from the stigma that addiction is dirty and other people will think poorly of you. Heroin addiction is a disease, and it needs to be treated that way. Gather the facts about the addiction, and waste no time in getting help for your addiction. If you are a family member of an addict, act quickly. Life has far too much beauty in it to waste it on the horrors of a heroin addiction. You are worth much more than that.

YOUR DECLARATION IS: *I will face this heroin addiction head-on. I will waste no time getting help and do what I can to beat it!*

ONWARD

Cocaine is another powerfully addictive drug that can consume a person's essence and bring their family members to their knees. In the next chapter, I examine cocaine use and addiction. I will discuss the personality changes that occur as the addiction progresses, the damage to the body, and its long-term effects on the life of the user and those close to them.

◇◇◇◇◇◇◇◇◇◇◇

CHAPTER 7

Cocaine—
Powerful Surrender

Cocaine makes you think you can conquer the world as it destroys your soul.

PROCESSES TO EMPLOY: Brutal Honesty, I Over E, Present-Understand-Fix, Slowing Down Life's Pace, Internal Focus, Fact-Finding, Honesty, Patience, Truth-Telling, Belief, Listening, Trust

---

COCAINE IS YET ANOTHER HIGHLY ADDICTIVE DRUG that produces powerful euphoric effects. Cocaine addicts love this drug for its hallucinogenic effects, speed kick, and the adrenaline rush they receive upon using the drug. This combination produces a false sense of confidence, convincing the user that they are powerful, can do anything they put their mind to, and nothing can stop them.

Cocaine is a tropane alkaloid that acts as a central nervous system stimulant. It is mainly used recreationally for its euphoric and rewarding effects. The action of cocaine impacts the nervous system by providing a powerful stimulant effect. This increases all the functions in the body, including neurological functioning. When using the drug, the user feels a euphoric reaction that adds a heightened sense of pleasure to the physical and intellectual acceleration.

Emotions are also heightened during cocaine use. Cocaine addicts will be highly reactive, and prone to aggression and violence. The combination of intense euphoria and physical and mental stimulation creates extreme impulsivity, with few, if any, pangs of conscience. People who abuse cocaine, and particularly those who become addicted to it, do what they want to do when they want to do it and how they want to do it. They have little, if any, concern for the feelings of others.

Withdrawal from cocaine includes many of the physical effects, intellectual confusion, and heightened emotions experienced with other drugs. Still, this drug's withdrawal also produces a steep drop in confidence and a sense of reduced power. When this happens, cocaine addicts feel stripped of their drug-induced powerful identity and will do anything to restore those feelings.

THE STATISTICS

Here are recent statistics regarding cocaine:[6]

➤ Among people aged twelve or older, in 2021, 1.7% (or about 4.8 million people) reported using cocaine in the past twelve months.

➤ In 2022, an estimated 0.5% of eighth graders, 0.3% of tenth graders, and 1.5% of twelfth graders reported using cocaine in the past twelve months.

➤ Among people aged twelve or older, in 2021, 0.5% (or about 1.4 million people) had a cocaine use disorder in the past twelve months in 2023.

➤ In 2021, approximately 24,486 people died from an overdose involving cocaine.

➤ Heart attack is the leading cause of death among people who abuse cocaine. One report shows it accounts for 25 percent of deaths among people ages eighteen to forty-five who have abused cocaine or crack cocaine.

THE PROGRESSION

1. The person is approached by others who use cocaine to give it a try, usually at a party or other social gathering.

2. After repeated coercion by others, the person agrees to try the drug.

3. The first experience is to either snort the drug or smoke it, depending on the availability.

4. The person likes the experience and considers doing it again.

5. The person decides to use the drug occasionally, perhaps as an addiction to other substances they use to "party."

6. The user now includes cocaine as a social-partying drug that can be used with other drugs like alcohol and marijuana.

7. The user begins to include cocaine in their typical partying environment. They usually use cocaine almost every time they party and begin to look forward to doing so. It is still used only occasionally.

8. The user likes the effects and progresses from snorting to smoking the drug as a routine way to administer it.

9. The drug is no longer used occasionally, and the user begins to use it as often as possible.

10. The addict now begins to accept cocaine as a "normal" part of their life.

11. The addict uses the drug every time it is available and does whatever is necessary to obtain it.

12. The addict's personality is changing; they firmly believe they are more powerful and the drug is a necessary part of their life.

13. The addict begins to make cocaine the most important part of life while family, friends, and important responsibilities are neglected.

14. The addict experiences withdrawal from the drug and now will do whatever they can to avoid that pain.

15. The addict begins stealing, robbing, selling the drug, and doing whatever they can to get high, regardless of the repercussions.

16. The addiction is in full swing.

Though the step-by-step progression may seem lengthy, cocaine addiction can occur quickly. The combination of euphoria and physical and emotional acceleration produces a high that makes the user feel invincible. For some people, addiction can occur after just a few experiences with the drug, while for others, the weekend routine and sporadic use can continue for an extended period.

Not all users experience the same high, and not all users progress through the steps the same way. In this way, cocaine is no different from any other drug. The effects of any drug are based on a person's individual physiology and environment. Also, different people will experience the damage cocaine causes in different ways. They will progress through the stages of use to abuse to addiction depending on their circumstances.

Cocaine addiction moves fast, and if the user has preexisting mental health issues, it can become dangerous quickly. Cocaine users are impulsive and can act without concern for others and any potential repercussions. They firmly believe that their way is the right way, can exhibit strong narcissistic tendencies, and can become aggressive and, at times, violent when they do not get their way.

IN THE CLUTCHES

No addiction is free from the problems and side effects that develop from continued use. What follows is a list of the effects that one can experience from addiction to any drug or activity. Different addictions can lead to different problems, as you will see as we continue.

PHYSICAL PROBLEMS—Immediate side effects from cocaine and crack cocaine include elevated blood pressure, rapid heartbeat, vasoconstriction in the brain and throughout the body, blood clots (which can lead to heart attack, pulmonary embolism, stroke, and deep vein thrombosis), angina (chest pain from tightening of the vessels), myocardial infarction (the death of heart muscle from lack of oxygen related to poor blood flow), permanently increased blood pressure, tachycardia (fast heart rate), and arrhythmia (irregular heart rate).

Snorting cocaine causes direct damage to the mucous membranes in the nose. With drier environments and less blood flow, the soft tissues in the nose will become damaged and eventually die. This will expose the cartilage lining between nasal cavities, known as the septum. Snorting cocaine can cause mucous membrane damage through the sinus cavity that leads to the throat and upper respiratory system. It constricts the blood vessels in the lungs. It destroys the alveolar walls so oxygen does not enter the bloodstream and causes the destruction of the capillaries that carry oxygen to the rest of the body. Chronic cough, higher risk of infections like pneumonia and tuberculosis, acute respiratory distress, asthma, and pulmonary edema are all associated with freebasing cocaine. People who chronically abuse crack cocaine can develop "crack lung" (eosinophilic pneumonitis).

MENTAL HEALTH ISSUES—These changes include paranoia, depression, anxiety, panic attacks, and cocaine psychosis (with symptoms such as delusions and hallucinations). Chronic cocaine users lose gray brain matter at a significantly faster rate, a sign of premature aging. The parts of the brain containing the most gray matter help control muscular and sensory activity, higher learning, attention, memory, thought, motor control, and coordination. The loss of gray matter has also been associated with bipolar disorder, schizophrenia, and Alzheimer's disease.

COMMUNICATION PROBLEMS—With the significant increase in physical, intellectual, and emotional energy, speech patterns are often accelerated, fragmented, and intense. While on the drug, addicts can become argumentative, impulsive, and overly focused on one particular thought. They have difficulty listening to others' opinions, tend to dominate conversations, and will instigate disagreements.

LEGAL PROBLEMS—Legal problems include aggravated assaults, physical and verbal violence, possession and other drug charges, burglaries, home invasions, and, in more drastic cases, murder.

FINANCIAL CONCERNS—Cocaine addicts will quickly use all available finances to obtain the drug. They are very impulsive and have a difficult time planning for future needs. They will use whatever resources are available to them at any given time to obtain what they want.

FAMILY AND RELATIONSHIP ISSUES—With the decrease in communication skills, combined with their propensity for violence, as well as their impulsive and single-minded approach to living, they have a difficult time maintaining relationships. They are routinely overly emotional, and their anger can accelerate within seconds. Family members tend to keep their distance.

EMPLOYMENT PROBLEMS—On mild doses of cocaine, people report that they can think more clearly and perform tasks more efficiently. However, as the drug begins to take over their lives, they cannot stay in one place for long, cannot focus on one task, have difficulty taking orders and working with other people, and are irresponsible concerning daily schedules. They often have a difficult time staying employed.

CHANGES IN SOCIAL LIFE—At lower doses of the drug, users find themselves more social and gregarious and enjoy being with other people, but as the addiction takes control, their quick reactions, emotional responses, and, at the very least, verbal abuse, pushes people away. They begin to associate almost exclusively with other drug users.

LYING—Consistent with all other drug users, cocaine users will rarely tell the truth about their use, what they are spending, who they are spending time with, where they are going, and about almost anything else that might threaten their ability to keep using the drug.

ACCOUNTABILITY ISSUES—When people use cocaine sporadically, they often report increased motivation and a willingness to get things done. They can be accountable at this level, but as the addiction progresses, they are unable to remain accountable consistently. People and responsibilities in their lives tend to be discounted as the addiction progresses.

PERSONALITY CHANGES—Cocaine addicts are demanding, temperamental, and can have difficulty connecting with the feelings of other people. They will experience paranoia, believe other people are out to get them, and become overly defensive about other people's intentions and their safety. They may experience intense and highly changeable moods, view things only in extremes (all good or all bad), and participate in impulsive and sometimes dangerous activities such as spending sprees, unsafe sex, reckless driving, binge eating, self-harm (cutting), inappropriate fits of anger, intense feelings of dissociation, and thoughts or threats of suicide.

ANGER AND VIOLENCE—Since the drug causes such a drastic increase in neurological functioning, and since the body is experiencing an enhanced fight-or-flight response, anger will be more prevalent, as will violence. At times, they will physically harm others.

COLLATERAL DAMAGE

In addition to the damage that cocaine does to the addict, it has a drastic effect on the way family members feel and the dynamics within the family. Family members will feel as though they are constantly walking on eggshells since even the slightest change in normal family operations can instigate reactions from addicts that range from minor verbal abuse to outright physical attacks.

Cocaine addicts will often damage property, steal from other family members, and behave in a fashion that has the characteristics of a borderline personality disorder. Their paranoia consistently puts family members in a defensive position as the addict accuses them of everything—from plotting against them to making threats and trying to hurt them. There will be financial loss, an impact on social relationships, legal problems that must be addressed, and dealing with hospitalizations and incarcerations. There's also the shame and guilt experienced by loved ones because they are not doing enough to help the addict fix it or fear they may be part of the problem.

Since cocaine causes so many physical problems, overdoses are always anticipated, and family members live in constant fear about what will happen on any given day. After a time, the health of the addict's loved ones can become compromised due to the anxiety and depression that result from being unable to help the addict or deal with their abuse.

These issues decrease physical and emotional health, and the addict's loved ones may experience difficulty focusing and being efficient. It is not uncommon for family members to seek help for medical issues and counseling and support services to help them address the changes they are personally experiencing.

SUMMING IT UP

Unlike its heroin counterpart, what happens with cocaine is fast and furious. Cocaine addicts live in an intense and highly accelerated world. They operate at a pace that causes abrupt and drastic changes to themselves and everyone they touch. There is no compromising with a cocaine addict. They see the world in black and white and assume everyone else will cooperate with their unrealistic desires.

Cocaine turns the world on hyperdrive. However, it is a physical, emotional, and intellectual state that can only last for short periods. The drug has to be used many times a day to keep the high constant. The expenses for cocaine can far exceed other drugs, and the effect it has on those who use it can quickly move from a heightened sense of euphoria to the point of devastating aggression.

If you or someone close to you is struggling with a cocaine addiction, seek help immediately. Call the National Drug Helpline at (844) 289-0879. It is free and confidential.

 TIME TO TAKE ACTION

1. Become as knowledgeable as you can about cocaine and cocaine addiction. The more information you have, the better equipped you are to deal with this potentially devastating problem.

2. If you either feel that you are addicted to cocaine or that it is causing significant problems in your life, waste no time and contact your primary care physician, go to an emergency room, or call the national drug helpline number above.

3. Cocaine addiction moves fast, and the treatment for it cannot wait. If you are suffering from cocaine addiction or know someone who is, waste no time and either make the call to the National Drug Helpline or get the addict to an emergency room.

4. Never walk on eggshells with a cocaine addict. This does nothing but keep the addiction strong. If you have a family member who is addicted, waste no time getting help from a physician, substance abuse professional, or a Narcotics Anonymous member to help you devise a plan to deal with the addiction.

5. As with all addictions, do not keep it a secret. There is nothing to be gained from hiding the fact that someone close to you is addicted. Talk to people you trust, and get help fast.

6. Part of dealing with cocaine addiction is to be in "protection mode." Protect your valuables and yourself. Keep this in mind. It is better to call the police in potentially violent situations than it is to attempt to hide the problem. Cocaine addiction is nothing to be fooled with.

7. Talk about the problem. Addiction counselors can help, and so can support people like Narcotics Anonymous. Al-Anon meetings are a good source of support for family members, or you can use the national abuse hotline.

 DRIVING IT HOME

There are no positive outcomes with cocaine addiction except recovery. This is a no-nonsense addiction that moves quickly and can devastate just as quickly. Be willing to treat a cocaine addict with warm but no-nonsense love. If you are the addict, try to stay away from the defenses and the games you play to keep your addiction active. Be willing to get the help you need. If you are a family member or someone close to them, let the addict know that you will not tolerate their aggressive behavior, and if necessary, back that up with law-enforcement personnel. Your best ally in the fight against cocaine addiction is to build a support and protection network that helps you avoid the damage cocaine can cause you and gives you the best opportunity to help the person who is addicted.

YOUR DECLARATION IS: *I will tackle cocaine addiction head-on. I will do what I must to stop it!*

 ONWARD

In the next chapter, I examine amphetamines and other stimulants. I will look at prescription medications, street drugs, and over-the-counter accelerants. I will discuss how life changes by abusing these substances and both the long and short-term effects physically, emotionally, and intellectually.

◇◇◇◇◇◇◇◇◇◇◇◇

CHAPTER 8

Amphetamines— The Real Speed Demon

They are the epitome of going nowhere fast. In the end, they leave you empty, exhausted, and burned out.

PROCESSES TO EMPLOY: Brutal Honesty, I Over E, Present-Understand-Fix, Slowing Down Life's Pace, Internal Focus, Fact-Finding, Honesty, Patience, Truth-Telling, Belief, Listening, Trust

---

AMPHETAMINES ARE STIMULANT DRUGS that accelerate messages between the brain and body. Doctors prescribe some amphetamines to treat conditions such as attention deficit hyperactivity disorder (ADHD), narcolepsy (an uncontrollable urge to sleep), and obesity. Other types, such as methamphetamine, are illegally produced and sold.

Methamphetamine, also a stimulant, is an illicit street drug that has no medical usage. Methamphetamine is often called by its street names like meth, crank, and ice. Consumed by injection, snorting, or smoking, this illicit synthetic stimulant is composed of amphetamine mixed with a variety of household substances. Drain cleaner, battery acid, paint thinner, or lighter fluid—all highly toxic to the human body—may all be used in the production of methamphetamine. The body has difficulty processing the ingredients used to produce methamphetamine, which can cause harsh psychological and physical effects.

The 2015 National Survey on Drug Use and Health (NSDUH) reports that about 4.8 million people in the United States abused prescription amphetamine medications that year, equivalent to about

1.8 percent of the population aged twelve and older. Prescription amphetamines include Adderall, Concerta, Dexedrine, Focalin, Metadate, Methylin, Ritalin, and Vyvanse.

Amphetamine statistics make it clear that more people are using these drugs than ever. Some studies published in the *National Library of Medicine* note that, from 2006 to 2016, there was a 2.5-fold increase in the use of these drugs in the United States. In 2006, 7.9 tons of the drugs were used, while in 2012, use peaked at 19.4 tons. By 2016, it had fallen to 18.6 tons. https://fherehab.com/amphetamine/statistics/#:~:-text=Statistics%20on%20Amphetamine%20Use&text=Some%20stud-ies%2C%20published%20in%20the,uses%20peaked%20at%2019.4%20tons.

THE STATISTICS

Here are some recent statistics regarding amphetamines:[7]

➤ Youth are more likely to abuse prescription stimulants than they are to abuse cocaine or amphetamines.

➤ 8.9% of eighth graders have tried amphetamines in their lifetime.

➤ 1.1% of eighth graders have tried methamphetamine.

➤ Eighth graders in 2020 are 56.1% more likely than 2017's eighth graders to have tried amphetamines.

➤ 4.4% of twelfth graders have used Adderall, while 4.3% have used amphetamine.

➤ 1.7% of twelfth graders use Ritalin, while 1.4% have used methamphetamine.

Like cocaine, amphetamine abuse and addiction can occur quickly. It is used in smaller doses to increase focus, motivation, clarity of thought, and energy. As the body and mind develop tolerance and an affinity for the drug, larger doses are used, and the addictive process does not take long to develop. Since the progression for prescription medications is a bit different, I will present its progression separately. The progression from use to abuse of methamphetamines is similar to what I presented for cocaine in Chapter 7.

THE PROGRESSION—
PRESCRIPTION-BASED AMPHETAMINES

1. Use begins by either obtaining a prescription for medication from a physician for a physical problem or using someone else's prescription either for a problem or experimentation.

2. If the initial use was from a physician, the prescription may be extended, and dependence may develop after two to four weeks of use.

3. If the initial use was someone else's prescription, and the person liked the effects, they may continue to use or try to get their own prescription.

4. The user will continue to use the prescription medication either as directed or until the supply runs out and tolerance for the drug increases and they begin to experience withdrawal effects.

5. The user will attempt to secure more medication either by trying to have their prescription extended further, by stealing someone else's prescription, or by beginning to purchase the drugs from friends and street-level dealers.

6. No longer able to secure the medication through their physician or someone else's prescription, they will seek out those who deal the drugs illegally.

7. Drugs will now be purchased regularly with the amount and type of drug depending on the need of the user.

8. As funds begin to become problematic, the addict will start stealing from family and friends to finance the habit.

9. As they understand what is happening, they protect their finances, and the addict begins to steal and sell their personal property and the property of family members and friends.

10. Shoplifting can become routine and, in some cases, can result in criminal charges.

11. At times, aggressive and violent behavior can begin, resulting in more serious crimes such as burglary, home invasions, and robbery.

THE PROGRESSION—METHAMPHETAMINES

12. The person is approached by others who use meth to give it a try, usually at a party or other social gathering.

13. After repeated coercion by others, the person agrees to try the drug.

14. The first experience is to snort the drug.

15. The person likes the experience and considers doing it again.

16. The person decides to use the drug occasionally as another way to "party."

17. The user now includes meth as a social partying drug that can be used with other drugs like alcohol and marijuana.

18. The user begins to include meth in their normal partying environment. It is still used only occasionally.

19. The user likes the effects and progresses from snorting to smoking the drug as a routine way to administer it.

20. The drug is no longer used occasionally, and the user begins to use it as often as possible.

21. The addict now begins to accept meth as a "normal" part of their life.

22. The addict uses the drug every time it is available and does whatever is necessary to obtain it.

23. The addict's personality is changing, and the drug has become a necessary part of their life.

24. The addict begins to make methamphetamine the most important

part of life, while family, friends, and important responsibilities are neglected.

25. The addict experiences withdrawal from the drug and now will do whatever they can to avoid that pain.

26. The addict begins stealing, robbing, selling the drug, and doing whatever they can to get high, regardless of the repercussions.

27. The addiction is in full swing.

Often, people who become addicted to amphetamines have either taken over-the-counter products, used stimulants like caffeine, stackers, and energy drinks, or have had prescriptions for conditions like ADD and ADHD, narcolepsy, or weight-loss issues. Some physicians have even prescribed them in small doses to help people with lethargy. Though addiction is not noticeable in lower doses, those who take these medications routinely do come to rely on them. They will notice the difference quickly if they miss a dose or run out.

Many people think that if a physician prescribes the medication, they will not become addicted. If taken as prescribed, the likelihood of addiction is reduced, and the more serious problems can be avoided. However, dependence on these drugs happens quickly, and like any drug, taken over time, the side effects can become more serious and cause prolonged physical, emotional, and intellectual damage. This does not mean you should not take an amphetamine-based medication if you have a problem that requires medicinal treatment. I am simply advising that if you are taking a medication that has amphetamine properties, it is very important to stay in touch with your physician, report any side effects or issues with dependency, and make adjustments if and when necessary.

Street drugs are an entirely different story. Methamphetamine has no medicinal value whatsoever, and the ingredients used to make it can have serious side effects and cause damage to your body, emotions, and mind that may, in time, be irreversible. Since there is no monitoring program available, such as is the case with prescription medications, the body will develop a tolerance quickly, and the abuse potential is significantly enhanced. Also, the root of delivery is often different from street drugs. Where almost all amphetamine-based pharmaceuticals are taken orally and in prescribed doses, street drugs may be taken orally, snorted, smoked, and injected. When one chooses to smoke crack or inject amphetamines, the effects are sudden, and the impact on the body and mind is dramatically more intense. Unfortunately, so is the damage it does.

IN THE CLUTCHES

No addiction is free from the problems and side effects that develop from continued use. What follows is a list of the effects that one can experience from addiction to any drug or activity. Different addictions can lead to different problems, as you will see as we continue.

PHYSICAL PROBLEMS—These issues include skin sores, chronic insomnia, sudden weight loss, high-risk behavior, hyperactivity, sagging skin, severe tooth decay, elevated blood pressure, rapid heartbeat, and vasoconstriction in the brain and throughout the body. Snorting methamphetamine can cause mucous membrane damage through the sinus cavity, leading to the throat and upper respiratory system. Blood vessels in the lungs constrict; alveolar walls are destroyed so oxygen does not enter the bloodstream; and capillaries that carry oxygen to the rest of the body can be destroyed. There is also a serious impact on the skeletal system and the muscles in the body as both remain tense for extended periods.

MENTAL HEALTH ISSUES—These issues include paranoia, nervous or anxious behavior, irritability, depression, anxiety, and panic attacks with symptoms such as delusions and hallucinations and, in extreme cases, psychosis.

COMMUNICATION PROBLEMS—With the significant increase in physical, intellectual, and emotional energy, speech patterns are often accelerated, fragmented, and intense. While on the drug, addicts can become argumentative, impulsive, and overly focused on one particular thought. They have a difficult time listening to the opinions of others and tend to dominate conversations and instigate disagreements.

LEGAL PROBLEMS—As the addiction progresses and the need for the drug increases, the addict can find themselves in altercations with others, some of which will be violent and result in arrest. Other times, they may be arrested for assault, burglary, theft, receiving stolen property, possession of controlled substances, and shoplifting. These charges may lead to fines, probation, and incarceration.

FINANCIAL CONCERNS—As the addiction progresses, much of the finances are used to support the addiction, and this can drain their resources and those of family members. Bills are left unpaid, the addict and family members may be subjected to calls from collection services, and in some cases, bankruptcy is filed.

FAMILY AND RELATIONSHIP ISSUES—Regardless of the etiology of the addiction, family relationships can quickly suffer. The addict is often angry, noncompliant, steals from family members, and brings negative attention to everyone associated with them. They will use family members and hurt them if necessary to secure the drug. Family relationships often are strained to the point of estrangement.

EMPLOYMENT PROBLEMS—In the early stages of the addiction, users can maintain employment and, at times, even be seen as very productive. As the addiction progresses, however, they will miss work, become argumentative, have a difficult time following directions, and have altercations with others in the workplace. This aggressive behavior often results in termination.

CHANGES IN SOCIAL LIFE—As the addiction progresses, the addict will sever relationships with friends, be aggressive with them, and be seen as people who are difficult to get along with. In the early stages, they are perceived as fun-loving and gregarious. It is in the later stages that the anger develops, and friendships become casualties.

LYING—The lying begins as the progression to addiction continues. As the user begins to use more of the drug, they will lie about their usage, where they are going when they are buying their drugs, how much they are using, who they are spending time with, and anything that might threaten the continued use of the drug. Lying becomes a way of life.

ACCOUNTABILITY ISSUES—In the early stages, when a person is becoming dependent on amphetamines, their energy and focus will increase, and they will seem highly accountable. However, as the addiction progresses, accountability will decrease, and they will be difficult to depend on. Even when they are there to help, they will be argumentative, want things their way, and engage in verbal and sometimes physical battles.

PERSONALITY CHANGES—Amphetamine addict's personality changes mirror those of cocaine addicts. They are demanding, temperamental, and have difficulty connecting with other people's feelings. They will experience paranoia, believe other people are out to get them, and become overly defensive about other people's intentions and their safety. They may experience intense and highly changeable moods, view things only in extremes (all good or all bad), participate in impulsive and sometimes dangerous activities such as spending sprees, unsafe sex, reckless driving, binge-eating, self-harm (cutting), inappropriate fits of anger, intense feelings of dissociation, and thoughts or threats of suicide.

ANGER AND VIOLENCE—The propensity for anger and violence always increases when someone is under the influence of amphetamines. In the early stages, the increase is minimal, usually limited to temperamental and impatient behavior. As the addiction progresses, they may be demanding, insolent, intolerant of others, and ready to strike quickly. When this happens, anger can quickly develop into violent behavior.

COLLATERAL DAMAGE

Even though it progresses fast, amphetamine addiction can sneak up on family members. When the medication comes from a family physician, family members will assume there should be no problems associated with using it. A doctor prescribes and monitors it; any problems can be dealt with before they cause issues in a person's life. This is not always the case.

Methamphetamine addiction can begin even under the care of qualified medical personnel.

Regardless of whether they are prescribed by a family physician or a person who purchases them from a drug dealer, when the use progresses to the stage of addiction, many of the symptoms are the same. The collateral damage (that is, the effects the addict never thought about) will become exacerbated and, at times, can be devastating. What started as a fun-loving joyride or a medication to treat a condition has turned into something that has caused serious complications for the person taking the drug and their loved ones.

Family members can be exposed to significant changes in the physical and mental health of the addicted person, may experience the loss of finances and property, and at times may be on the receiving end of their anger and violence. It is not uncommon for family members to be faced with either having their addicted family member arrested or removing them from their home. At times, their safety may be at risk.

SUMMING IT UP

It is always difficult to report a family member for aggressive behavior, but it is also difficult to be a part of the roller-coaster ride through the addict's addiction. There may come a time when family members may need to get together to make decisions about how they are going to deal with the addict. Amphetamine addicts are often resistant to treatment, and treatment for the addiction usually follows either a period of incarceration or some other crisis. If you think amphetamines may be affecting your life, and you find it difficult to stop using them, you should call your primary care physician to make an appointment or get yourself to the closest emergency room.

If you or someone close to you is suffering from amphetamine addiction, call the National Drug Helpline at (844) 289-0879. It is free and confidential.

1. For those who may be having problems with amphetamines: If you feel you are having a problem with an amphetamine-based drug, talk to your physician or an addiction counselor to help you begin the process of recovery.

2. For family members: Talk to your physician and your pharmacist. Get as much information as you can about prescription medications and methamphetamine. Knowing the facts is the foundation for efficient action.

3. Make a list of the hospitals, support programs, and treatment facilities that can assist in the recovery from amphetamine abuse and addiction. You will need this to implement a treatment plan for the addict.

4. Have a plan in place if you feel that someone in your family has a problem with amphetamines. The time to execute that plan may come sooner than you think.

5. Talk about the problem. Addiction counselors can help, and so can support people like Narcotics Anonymous. Al-Anon meetings are good for family members, or you can use the national abuse hotline.

 DRIVING IT HOME

Amphetamine addiction moves quickly. It can kill the addict and destroy families. If you are addicted to amphetamines or believe you have a serious problem with them, there is always help for those who are willing to do what it takes to recover from the effects of a drug that can shatter your world. No one fights an addiction alone. There is always help available. The recovery plan takes work, and it is not easy, but it is also not impossible. Your life is worth far more than what an addiction has to offer. Family is always more important than a drug. Get the help you need to begin a recovery program that can change the rest of your life. You deserve to be happy.

YOUR DECLARATION IS: *I will get help for my amphetamine addiction. I will do what it takes to remove this life-threatening nemesis from my world!*

 ONWARD

In the next chapter, I examine hallucinogens. I will look at today's medical model and how some physicians are beginning to prescribe them for medical issues. I will also look at street-level hallucinogens, what they do to the user emotionally and intellectually, the hallucinogenic experience, and the long-term effects of continued hallucinogenic abuse.

CHAPTER 9

Hallucinogens— From Fantasy to Nightmare

They are a mirage, showing you the colors of the rainbow. When used without guidance, they can turn your brain to mush.

PROCESSES TO EMPLOY: Brutal Honesty, I Over E, Present-Understand-Fix, Slowing Down Life's Pace, Internal Focus, Fact-Finding, Honesty, Patience, Truth-Telling, Belief, Listening, Trust

---

HALLUCINOGENS ARE AMONG THE OLDEST KNOWN GROUP of drugs used for their ability to alter human perception and mood. The most commonly abused hallucinogens, such as psilocybin-containing mushrooms, LSD, and MDMA (ecstasy), are typically taken orally or smoked. Hallucinogens are a classification of drugs that alter the user's perception of reality.

Psilocybin (magic mushrooms) is a hallucinogenic substance found in certain types of mushrooms. Acid, also known as lysergic acid diethylamide (LSD), is a synthetic hallucinogen. It is typically a white powder or clear liquid. Mescaline (peyote) is a hallucinogenic substance found in some types of cactuses, including the peyote cactus. Peyote has traditionally been used in certain Native American spiritual rituals. Ecstasy, also known as MDMA, is a synthetic hallucinogen and stimulant. Phencyclidine (PCP) is a hallucinogenic drug that creates the feeling of being separated from your body and surroundings. PCP is commonly known as angel dust.

MDMA and dissociative hallucinogen drugs like PCP are more addictive on a neurobiological level due to the changes the drugs create in the brain. Hence, young adults who have used these drugs for an extended period can experience withdrawal symptoms after they stop using. Hallucinogen use disorder, which can result from chronic overuse of a hallucinogen, is more likely to produce compulsive behaviors and psychological dependence than physical addiction.

The primary action of hallucinogenic drugs is on the brain and nervous system. Though they do alter perception and mood, changing the way the brain perceives and interprets information, addiction to these drugs is primarily neurological. Though there are reports of some physical addiction, this is seen as secondary to the neurological transitions.

THE STATISTICS

Here are some recent statistics regarding hallucinogens:[8]

➤ Hallucinogenic drug use has increased among American adults aged twenty-six and over, with over 5.5 million people using psychedelic substances in 2019.

➤ Since 2015, psychedelic drug use has increased overall—particularly among adults twenty-six and older—but decreased in adolescents aged twelve to seventeen years, according to a new study by Columbia University Mailman School of Public Health and Columbia University Irving Medical Center.

➤ In 2019 alone, over 5.5 million people in the United States used hallucinogens. In 2002, 1.7% of the population over the age of twelve took a hallucinogen in a given year, whereas in 2019, this rose to 2.2%.

➤ One in every twelve young adults and more than one in ten college students use hallucinogenic drugs.

➤ In the past decade, ending in 2023young adult hallucinogen use has nearly tripled.

➤ The use of LSD has been relatively stable among young adults in recent years, remaining around 4 percent. However, the number of young adults using non-LSD hallucinogens, such as psilocybin and PCP, doubled from 2018 to 2021 (from 3.4% to 6.6 %). MDMA (also called ecstasy or Molly) is the only hallucinogen that showed a significant decrease in use during the same period.

With the advent of the legalization of marijuana and research regarding the use of hallucinogenic substances in the treatment of mental health disorders, many young people no longer perceive these drugs as dangerous. The use of hallucinogens in mental health treatment is closely monitored, and the patient's psychological and medical history are factored into the program. Any negative results are noted and can be quickly addressed by the medical team. Also, those who are administering the drug are trained professionals.

When people use hallucinogens in recreational settings, the dangerous side effects can be more pronounced since there is no monitoring protocol to address any negative reactions. Not all hallucinogenic experiences are positive. Though "bad trips" are in the vast minority, they can have a devastating effect on a person's brain and neurology when they are severe. People also mix hallucinogenic drugs with other drugs, particularly alcohol and marijuana. In some cases, hallucinogens are mixed with amphetamines such as MDMA. This can cause a person to act on the false reality created by the hallucinogenic drugs.

The effects of hallucinogenic drugs depend on the type of drug being used, the strength of the dose of the drug, and the individual characteristics of the person taking them. These characteristics include age, sex, biology, medical history, mental health, and mood. When a person is angry, depressed, and anxious, their experience may reflect these feelings. However, better experiences are reported by those who are happy and relaxed when they take the drug.

The progression from use to abuse with hallucinogenic drugs is a bit different than with other drugs. Since there is minimal physical dependence, most withdrawal experienced will be on the intellectual or emotional level. One typically does not crave the drug on a physical level during periods of abstinence, and there are reduced physical withdrawal effects when compared to other drugs.

THE PROGRESSION

1. Typically, friends will offer the person the drug either at a party, social event, or in a small group.

2. The person will typically not use the drug when first offered, electing to think it over.

3. After some consideration, the person tries one of the hallucinogens for the first time. If the experience is enjoyable, a second experience is planned.

4. The person tries the hallucinogen for the second time and enjoys the experience.

5. The hallucinogen user now plans to use the drug more often, usually in the presence of other people.

6. As with other drugs, the user will be approached to try a different hallucinogen. The user accepts the offer.

7. The second hallucinogenic drug is tried, and the experience is enjoyed.

8. This leads to trying other hallucinogenic drugs.

9. For some, using the drug will remain sporadic, with use possibly on the weekends.

10. Pleasurable "trips" will be planned more often for others, especially those who need to escape reality or difficult circumstances.

11. As perceptions change and reality becomes skewed, the user begins to use the drug regularly. This could be done several times per week and, in some cases, more often.

12. The addict uses the drug whenever available, as the psychological and emotional dependence becomes more significant.

13. As neurological changes become more pronounced, the addict depends on the drug to restore their perception of a positive reality.

14. The addiction to the drug has taken hold, and the realistic circumstances in one's life are replaced by those created in the drug-induced states.

As the user progresses from sporadic use to emotional and intellectual addiction, reality becomes distorted, and the need to restore the drug-induced version of reality is enhanced. Hallucinogen addicts report having a difficult time living without the drug as the neurological dependence increases. This is where the need for the drug begins to establish permanence and where the use of the drug can increase to many times per week and to daily use for some people.

Hallucinogen-persisting perception disorder can develop when someone experiences the effects of hallucinogens after the substance has physically left their system. These occurrences affect the minimum of hallucinogenic drug users, but when they do develop, they can quickly develop into extreme paranoia, neuroses, sustained perceptual difficulties, and, in some cases, psychosis. It is not out of the question for someone to commit suicide during a hallucinogenic experience or during a hallucinogen-persisting perception disorder when the drug is no longer in the system.

IN THE CLUTCHES

No addiction is free from the problems and side effects that develop from continued use. What follows is a list of the effects that one can experience from addiction to any drug or activity. Different addictions can lead to different problems, as you will see as we continue.

PHYSICAL PROBLEMS—Physiological effects include elevated heart rate, increased blood pressure, dizziness, nausea, dilated pupils, and disturbing visions. Hallucinogens can induce nausea and vomiting, abdominal pain, diarrhea, tremors, headache, lower or faster heart rate, and a sensation of "floating."

MENTAL HEALTH ISSUES—Using hallucinogens is associated with higher levels of anxiety, depression, PTSD, intense emotions that can range from bliss to fear, panic attacks, paranoia, confusion, alteration of mood and thoughts, a sense of detachment or dissociation, visions, hallucinations, and other changes in perception of reality.

COMMUNICATION PROBLEMS—With sporadic use, particularly in the early stages, there is little effect on communication when the person is not using the drug. Under the influence of a hallucinogenic drug, communication can be fragmented and unrealistic. With regular and continued use, even when the person is not using the drug, communication can remain fragmented and unrealistic.

LEGAL PROBLEMS—Legal problems regarding hallucinogenic drugs usually occur under the influence when behaviors can reflect perceptual changes and under the influence of some hallucinogenic drugs such as PCP and MDMA. Perceptions can become distorted, often leading to behaviors that are unrealistic and often dangerous. At times, users may act on irrational impulses, leading to arrests and criminal charges.

FINANCIAL CONCERNS—Financial concerns are not as intense as with other drugs; however, with sustained use and perceptible changes, users can have a difficult time maintaining employment, causing financial concerns. Also, with sustained use, costs for the drug increase and can impact the finances of the addict and their families.

FAMILY AND RELATIONSHIP ISSUES—With sporadic use, family relationships may become strained but not to the point of dysfunction. Family relationships can become increasingly strained with sustained use, especially when communication and rational thoughts diminish. In severe cases, psychosis can develop, exacerbating an already difficult situation.

EMPLOYMENT PROBLEMS—Employment issues are uncommon with sporadic use; however, with sustained use and perceptual changes, it is difficult to maintain focus and be dependable, which can cause problems in the workplace.

CHANGES IN SOCIAL LIFE—With sporadic use, there are no significant changes in one's social life. However, when hallucinogen use progresses to the point of addiction, friends will have a difficult time communicating with the addict. The addict's perception of reality will change, which makes it difficult to continue with normal social relationships.

LYING—Almost any drug involvement includes lying to some extent. Hallucinogenic users will lie if they are asked about using, but until it progresses to the point of addiction, lying is not a serious problem. When it does reach the point of addiction, however, lying increases, but the hold on reality changes, and the individual may not know fact from fiction.

ACCOUNTABILITY ISSUES—Accountability is usually not a problem in the early stages. However, as the addiction begins to control the addict's life, they become unfocused and undependable and have a difficult time staying with and completing tasks.

PERSONALITY CHANGES—Some users will become more introverted when using hallucinogenic drugs, while others will become more extroverted. There also tends to be an increase in introspective activity. Some people become more argumentative, while others become more open to different opinions. There seem to be no permanent personality changes with sporadic use. However, there is the danger of developing hallucinogenic personality disorder with sustained use.

ANGER AND VIOLENCE—Anger and violence can be expressed under the influence of a "bad trip." Also, with hallucinogenic drugs that have an amphetamine formula included in their composition, like MDMA, people may act out on impulsive and unrealistic perceptions. Some of those actions may include anger and violence.

COLLATERAL DAMAGE

Collateral damage regarding the use of hallucinogenic drugs is not usually as drastic as it is with drugs like cocaine, methamphetamine, and heroin. In the early stages of use, users can easily hide their use from family members and significant others. The drug is usually used outside of the home, and family members may be unaware that it has been part of the user's partying lifestyle for some time. However, there are times when someone can use the drug for the first time and experience psychotic effects. These are usually seen with more potent drugs like MDMA and PCP, though depending on the person's mental health and physiology, it could happen with any of the hallucinogens.

When the use becomes more frequent, the user's personality can change. When use becomes an addiction, family members may experience a notable disconnection in their relationship with the addict and in the way this person interacts with others. Even in cases where the addict remains close to family members, the quality of the relationship can deteriorate, and family members may struggle to make sense of the addict's actions and words.

With continued sporadic use, the perceptual changes in the user are usually minimal. However, with continued use, thoughts can become irrational, and the addict may firmly believe that the drug-induced reality is, in fact, actual reality. In these cases, it is difficult to predict the addict's behavior, and aggression and violence are possible. In extreme cases, family members could be severely injured or lose their lives to an addict who firmly believes the fantasy that the family member plans to hurt them or "someone" has told them to hurt the person for a perceived valid reason.

Aggression and violence aside, when the addiction progresses to the point of unrealistic thoughts and behaviors or psychosis, family members will find themselves in a position to try to rescue their sick family member. This may include police involvement, outpatient counseling, and, in more severe cases, hospitalization.

SUMMING IT UP

Hallucinogenic drugs are gaining popularity, particularly with younger people. The legalization of marijuana and the press coverage of possible therapeutic uses for hallucinogenic drugs have reduced the fear associated with the adverse effects of abusing these drugs. When this happens, people tend to take risks with drugs that have the potential to do severe intellectual and emotional damage in unmonitored situations. Under the right circumstances and strict supervision, hallucinogens may eventually be prescribed to treat disorders like PTSD, depression, and anxiety. Until the research is conclusive and the proper protocols are in place, people must refrain from sustained use of these drugs.

If you feel that you are having a problem with hallucinogenic drugs, you can call the National Drug Helpline at (844) 289-0879. It is free and confidential.

 ## TIME TO TAKE ACTION

1. Hallucinogenic drugs are in a class of their own. Do the research and know everything you need to know about them. Get your information from credible sources.

2. The research about using hallucinogenic drugs to help with mental health concerns is still in its infancy. Wait for the results before you attempt to use these drugs.

3. If you are considering using hallucinogenic drugs therapeutically, do so only under the guidance of a person trained in this therapeutic treatment modality.

4. If you have taken hallucinogenic drugs and are experiencing perceptual changes that continue into your daily living when you are not using the drug, contact your primary-care physician immediately.

5. If your family member has been using hallucinogenic drugs or is exhibiting signs of unrealistic thoughts and actions, schedule a consultation with your primary care physician.

6. Chronic hallucinogenic drug users often exhibit irrational thinking. These thoughts may develop into actions that can be dangerous to others. Err, on the side of caution with this one, get help if you need it.

7. **Call the National Drug Helpline at (844) 289-0879. It is free and confidential.**

 ## DRIVING IT HOME

As the research into hallucinogenic drug therapy continues, it makes sense to take a step back until the research becomes more conclusive. Recreationally, using these drugs carries huge risks, and even though they are not as physically addictive as many other drugs, their ability to permanently change personality is always a potential and severe side effect. You should never attempt to change your perception of reality because you are dissatisfied with your life. The better advice is to make the changes that create happiness and productivity instead of infusing your world with a false sense of reality that may eventually betray you.

YOUR DECLARATION IS: *I will keep myself grounded in my own rational reality so I do not need to change it artificially!*

 ## ONWARD

In the next chapter, I will examine marijuana and its potential for addiction. I will discuss some of its positive medical effects and some of the more debilitating effects on the body and mind, and I will forecast the potentially serious side effects that may occur with continued use.

CHAPTER 10

Marijuana—The New Mind-Dulling Medicine

It is touted as the new medical savior. In the end, a drug is a drug, and they all come with a price.

PROCESSES TO EMPLOY: Brutal Honesty, I Over E, Present-Understand-Fix, Slowing Down Life's Pace, Internal Focus, Fact-Finding, Honesty, Patience, Truth Telling, Belief, Listening, Trust

---

IN THE EARLY 1900S, ALCOHOL WAS BEING CHAMPIONED as a cure-all. It was the elixir that could cure most problems people had. Today, marijuana has supplanted the world elixir as the new wonder drug. It is being used to lower blood pressure, reduce inflammation, treat anxiety disorders and depression, treat gastrointestinal (GI) disorders, prevent seizures, and even fight cancer.

Marijuana is a mind-altering psychoactive drug composed of a dry, shredded, green/brown mix of flowers, stems, seeds, and leaves from the *Cannabis sativa* plant. It goes by many street names: Aunt Mary, BC Bud, Blunt, Boom, Chronic, Dope, Gangster, Ganja, Grass, Hash, Herb, Hydro, Indo, Joint, Kif, Mary Jane, Mota, Pot, Reefer, Sinsemilla, Skunk, Smoke, Weed, and Yerba. The plant contains the low-grade mind-altering chemical THC (delta-9-tetrahydrocannabinol), an ingredient that produces the psychoactive effect, and other similar compounds. Marijuana is, by far, the most popular drug in America and arguably the most popular drug in the world.

Currently, forty of the fifty states have some form of marijuana legalization law on the books. Eight states—AK, CA, CO, MA, ME, NV, OR, WA, and the District of Columbia have legalized marijuana for recreational use. More than half of the states (twenty-nine) and the District of Columbia have legalized medical marijuana. An additional seventeen states allow the legal use of only limited CBD/low-THC marijuana for certain medical purposes. These numbers are expected to increase steadily.

THE STATISTICS

Here are some recent statistics regarding marijuana:[9]

➤ Approximately half of Americans, some 78 million people, claimed to have used marijuana at some point in their lifetime.

➤ Approximately 35 million Americans use marijuana every month.

➤ In 2023, 55 million Americans in total had reported using marijuana within the past year. This is higher than the number of active tobacco smokers, which is approximately 36.5 million, according to the Centers for Disease Control and Prevention (CDC).

➤ This means that there are 50.68% more marijuana users than there are tobacco smokers.

➤ Marijuana is the most commonly used federally illegal drug in the United States; 48.2 million people, or about 18% of Americans, used it at least once in 2019.

➤ Recent research estimated that approximately three in ten people who use marijuana have marijuana use disorder. For people who begin using marijuana before age eighteen, the risk of developing marijuana use disorder is even greater.

Marijuana use directly affects the brain, specifically the parts of the brain responsible for memory, learning, attention, decision-making, coordination, emotion, and reaction time. Infants, children, and teens (who still have developing brains) are especially susceptible to the adverse effects of marijuana.

One study has linked cannabis use to brain thinning in adolescents. This could significantly affect dendritic branching, a multi-step biological process by which neurons form new dendritic trees and branches to create new synapses. Activity taking place within the dendrites that branch off the neuron cell bodies is an important key to memory formation. See https://www.medscape.com/viewarticle/cannabis-use-linked-brain-thinning-adolescents-2024a1000k29?ecd=WNL_trdalrt_pos1_241108_etid6984585&uac=77912BK&impID=6984585

There are several ways to use marijuana. Some people smoke it in hand-rolled cigarettes (joints), in pipes, or water pipes (bongs). Others empty cigars and fill the shell with the drug (blunts). It is also mixed in food (edibles), such as brownies, cookies, or candy, or brewed in teas. Some users prefer the resins from marijuana, such as hash oil or honey oil (a gooey liquid), wax or budder (a soft solid with a texture like lip balm), or shatter (a hard, amber-colored solid). These extracts can deliver large amounts of THC to the body. This causes the user to feel the effects faster, with a "high" that is considerably more intense.

THE PROGRESSION

1. The initial use could be with family or friends, as part of a medical doctor's prescription, or in social settings.

2. During the first use, the person will experience the euphoria associated with the drug, and if they like the effects, they will continue to use the drug sporadically.

3. Some people may continue with sporadic use, while others will begin to use the drug more often, typically several times per week.

4. In states where medicinal marijuana has been approved, some people may secure medical cards to purchase the drug legally.

5. Some people will acquire medical cards but continue to purchase the drug from street sources as well as dispensaries.

6. For some, use will progress to smoking it daily.

7. The user begins to enjoy the euphoria and the relaxing effects of the drug and incorporates it into a regular part of their life.

8. For some, the use will remain daily, usually for periods of relaxation at the end of the day.

9. Others will use the drug several times per day for relaxation and the euphoric effects and to medicate conditions like anxiety and depression.

10. Some users will progress to the point that the drug is used several times a day. It may be smoked, vaped, or added to other food sources to produce marijuana edibles.

11. For these people, without their understanding, dependence on the drug is now developing.

12. The user believes that the drug is adding quality to their life and that continued use will increase their happiness and productivity.

13. Denial begins to set in, and the user, now becoming addicted to the drug, uses it routinely many times per day.

14. Now addicted to the drug, the addict is spending larger amounts of money on the drug, securing it from a variety of sources, and using it throughout the day.

15. When the drug is unavailable, or when only smaller amounts are available, demanding fewer uses, withdrawal effects are experienced, such as cravings, anxiety, restlessness, irritability, disturbed sleep and vivid dreams, gastrointestinal tract symptoms (for example, abdominal pain), night sweats, and tremors.

16. When the addict does not have the funds to purchase the drug at the level at which they are currently using it, withdrawal effects can include irritability, anger, hostility, headaches, body aches, and insomnia.

17. Now addicted to the drug, the addict makes sure that at all costs, they have uninterrupted possession of the drug to avoid the withdrawal effects.

IN THE CLUTCHES

No addiction is free from the problems and side effects that develop from continued use. What follows is a list of the effects that one can experience from addiction to any drug or activity. Different addictions can lead to different problems, as you will see as we continue.

PHYSICAL PROBLEMS—The issues can include altered senses (for example, seeing brighter colors), altered sense of time, changes in mood, impaired body movement, difficulty with thinking and problem-solving, impaired memory, hallucinations (when taken in high doses), delusions (when taken in high doses), psychosis (risk is highest with regular use of high-potency marijuana), and impaired brain development. At high doses, there may be nausea and vomiting. Using marijuana during pregnancy may increase the risk of pregnancy complications such as premature deliveries. Pregnant and breastfeeding women should avoid marijuana. Marijuana can raise the heart rate for up to three hours after smoking. This effect may increase the chance of heart attack. Older people and those with heart problems may be at higher risk. People who use vape pens are at risk for damage to the lungs and esophagus caused by the high levels of heat needed to produce the vapor.

MENTAL HEALTH ISSUES—Long-term marijuana use has been linked to mental illness in some people, such as hallucinations, paranoia, disorganized thinking, worsening symptoms in patients with schizophrenia, and increases in anxiety and depression for some people.

COMMUNICATION PROBLEMS—At lower doses, communication is only minimally affected. Most people tend to become more introverted when they use the drug and may communicate less often. Also, the content of communication typically remains at a more trivial level. People who are addicted to marijuana have a more difficult time organizing thoughts, and their communication is reflective of that.

LEGAL PROBLEMS—Legal problems are not considered significant with marijuana use. They usually result from possession of the drug in larger amounts, dealing the drug illegally, and, in some states, DUIs.

FINANCIAL CONCERNS—Financial concerns with marijuana occur less than with other drugs due to its legality, lower price, and availability. Financial problems may result from unemployment or issues unrelated directly to using the drug. At times, legal problems could create some financial stress.

FAMILY AND RELATIONSHIP ISSUES—Marijuana typically does not cause significant family problems. People may isolate themselves more often and are less motivated, leading to incomplete household tasks. More issues result from perceived laziness and an unwillingness to be part of the household responsibilities. However, problems can develop when the use progresses to an addiction. These may include financial concerns, communication issues, and longer periods of isolation.

EMPLOYMENT PROBLEMS—At lower doses, there is little effect on unemployment. When the use progresses to this stage of addiction, employees are unmotivated and experience focusing problems, which may result in termination. Also, at higher doses, there can be tardiness and absentee issues.

CHANGES IN SOCIAL LIFE—At lower doses, there are few, if any, changes to the user's social life. As the use progresses to the addictive phase, people may isolate, communicate less with others, and slowly not find social life as important as it once was.

LYING—Lying generally doesn't increase with marijuana use. Any diversions from the truth tend to be associated with responsibilities and accountability.

ACCOUNTABILITY ISSUES—At higher doses, it is difficult to depend on the marijuana addict. They typically make themselves unavailable to address responsibilities, may not focus enough to be accountable, and don't like their euphoria interrupted.

PERSONALITY CHANGES—Personality changes as a result of marijuana use tend to be minor. There is a reduction in motivation. People who regularly use cannabis may develop amotivation syndrome. This condition is marked by a low or nonexistent drive to engage in pleasurable activities and situations.

ANGER AND VIOLENCE—Anger or violence is rarely seen with marijuana use. However, during withdrawal from the drug, an individual could become angrier and possibly become violent.

COLLATERAL DAMAGE

Collateral damage is at a minimum with marijuana users at lower levels. Damage to the user comes from inhaling the smoke or vapor when using vape pens, chemicals that may be added to the marijuana, slower information-processing times, and reduced motivation. At higher doses, however, they may lose jobs and other employment opportunities, and their motivation issues may affect their productivity and their relationships.

Family members typically have issues with accountability and getting things done on time. At higher levels, marijuana users may not be up to date on their bills and can have many tasks that are either in need of attention or are waiting to be finished.

Communication within the family can suffer even at lower doses. Though the effect is minimal with sporadic use, with addictive use, there can be a significant impact on the quantity and quality of communication between family members and the reduced motivation and accountability that drugs can produce. There is no propensity for violence except in cases of acute withdrawal where an individual uses the drug often and in large amounts. This can produce withdrawal, which is far more intense.

SUMMING IT UP

Regardless of how the movement to legalize marijuana was framed, it is still a drug. All drugs have harmful side effects. Like many prescription drugs, marijuana does have some positive medicinal uses. It can relieve pain and discomfort in cancer patients, it can lower anxiety levels, and it can be used for chronic pain, to mention just a few. Conversely, acute cannabis toxicity results in difficulty with coordination, decreased muscle strength, reduced hand steadiness, postural hypotension (low blood pressure), lethargy, decreased concentration, slowed reaction time, slurred speech, and conjunctival injection (bloodshot eyes).

As marijuana continues to be legalized across the nation, the use of medical cards will be minimized as it will be available without prescriptions. It will fall into the category of a recreational drug, and we can expect its usage to continue to grow. As it does, we will continue to see some of the positive effects but expect the adverse effects listed earlier to rear their ugly heads more often. It is important to understand this before you decide to use the drug and how you intend to use it.

If you feel that you are having a problem with marijuana, you can call the National Drug Helpline at (844) 289-0879. It is free and confidential.

 TIME TO TAKE ACTION

1. The movement from medical marijuana to the legalization of marijuana didn't always provide the information people need to understand it. Take some time to gather as much information as you can about this drug, how it can benefit you, and what problems it may cause in your life.

2. Use marijuana only when necessary and as prescribed by your primary care physician or psychiatrist. Try not to make it something you do many times per day.

3. Be honest about your marijuana use. Like any other drug, people like to minimize their self-reports. Honesty can help you avoid the problems marijuana addiction can cause.

4. If you feel as though your marijuana use is beginning to affect your life in negative and unproductive ways, make an appointment with an addiction counselor to help you through these problems.

5. If you suspect a family member is becoming addicted to marijuana, it makes good sense to contact an addiction counseling professional to help you address the situation.

 ## DRIVING IT HOME

Regardless of how you choose to use it, marijuana is still a drug. Every drug has its side effects, and every drug can damage your body, your emotions, and your mind. The adverse effects are minimal when used as prescribed and in small doses; in higher doses, you can expect some of the physical, personality, and intellectual effects mentioned in this chapter. If you plan to use marijuana, do the research and understand everything you need to know about it. The rule is to use it in a way that benefits your life without it taking control of your world.

YOUR DECLARATION IS: *Marijuana is a drug, and I will be careful and knowledgeable regarding my use of it!*

 ## ONWARD

In the next chapter, I will examine food addiction. Though we need food to survive, when it is abused, it changes the way a person's mind, emotions, and body operate. I will be looking at self-image, body image, and the control-to-out-of-control cycle that develops when food becomes an addiction, and I will also be examining the relationship between food and bulimia and anorexia.

◇◇◇◇◇◇◇◇◇◇◇◇

CHAPTER 11

Food—The Wonder Drug

It is the embodiment of the double-edged sword. You need it to live,
but it could be the death of you.

PROCESSES TO EMPLOY: Brutal Honesty, I Over E, Present-
Understand-Fix, Slowing Down Life's Pace, Internal Focus, Fact-
Finding, Honesty, Patience, Truth-Telling, Belief, Listening, Trust

---

OF ALL THE SUBSTANCES AND ACTIVITIES A person can become addicted to, food is the most enigmatic of all. The human body needs it to survive, but when food is used improperly, it creates a whirlwind of harmful consequences. When we eat with nutrition in mind, paying attention to the types of food we are eating, the portion sizes, when we eat, and how fast we eat, food can keep us healthy, provide us with the energy we need, provide fuel for our brain, and supply every system in the body with what it needs to run efficiently.

However, when we incorporate unhealthy eating patterns into our lives, things can go awry quickly. Overeating can cause weight gain and lead to diabetes, heart disease, high blood pressure, high cholesterol, high triglyceride levels, and stomach and intestinal problems. Purging and not eating enough food can cause nutritional issues, leading to intellectual confusion, physical and emotional exhaustion, frequent illnesses, depression, and anxiety, to mention just a few consequences.

In this chapter, I will look at overeating and the obsessive need to prioritize food in unhealthy ways that can cause severe problems. I will also be looking at bulimia and anorexia as addictive processes and foods roll in maintaining them. Bulimia is an eating disorder in which a person has regular episodes of eating a huge amount of food (bingeing), during which the person feels a loss of control over their eating. The person then uses different ways to prevent weight gain, such as vomiting or laxatives (purging). Anorexia is an eating disorder characterized by restriction of food intake leading to low body weight, typically accompanied by intense fear of gaining weight and disturbed perception of body weight and image. Symptoms include trying to maintain a below-normal weight through starvation, laxatives, purging, or too much exercise.

THE STATISTICS—FOOD ADDICTION

Research from the University of Michigan showed the prevalence of food addiction by gender. For those suffering from food addictions, the following were reported:[10]

➤ 22% of women aged fifty to sixty-four and 18% of women aged fifty to eighty

➤ 32% of women who say their physical health is fair or poor

➤ 14% of men who say their physical health is fair or poor

➤ 45% of women who say their mental health is fair or poor

➤ 23% of men who say their mental health is fair or poor

➤ 17% of men who self-report they are overweight

➤ 34% of women who self-report they are overweight

➤ 51% of women who say they often feel isolated from others

➤ 26% of men say they often feel isolated from others

In discussing food addiction, it is important to note that two components must be addressed. The first is the food addiction. By this, I mean people who are addicted to food the same way other people are addicted to drugs. They have a difficult time regulating their consumption, and as a result, conditions like obesity and obsessive-compulsive eating develop. The second component is the control of food. People handle stress, insecurity, and other feelings in different ways. Sometimes, it may seem that the only way to control one's life is to control food intake.

There is eating to live, and there is living to eat...or not eat. Our bodies are thinking and acting machines that must be nurtured to operate efficiently. The formula is to put the right foods in our bodies in the right amounts. We provide our bodies with the vitamins and nutrients essential to healthy living, and we do our best to avoid unhealthy habits and ways of eating that can adversely affect our health. Those unhealthy habits can lead to life changes that range from mild to deadly, such as:

➤ Gorging on more food than one can physically tolerate

➤ Eating to the point of feeling ill

➤ Going out of the way to obtain certain foods

➤ Continuing to eat certain foods even if no longer hungry

➤ Eating in secret or in isolation

➤ Avoiding social interactions, relationships, or functions to spend time eating certain foods

➤ Difficulty functioning in a career or job due to decreased efficiency regarding the responsibilities of their job description.

➤ Spending a significant amount of money on buying certain foods for bingeing

➤ Decreased energy, chronic fatigue

➤ Difficulty concentrating

➤ Sleep disorders, such as insomnia or oversleeping

➤ Restlessness

➤ Irritability

➤ Headaches

➤ Digestive disorders

➤ Suicidal ideation

For some people, foods serve other purposes than nutrition, satisfying hunger, harmless munching, and attending celebratory dinners and events. For these people, food can serve as medicine, therapy, an escape from problems, a diversion from worry, a substitute for nurturance/ protection/safety, reward, punishment, and a coping mechanism. When food is used in this fashion, it can quickly become an addiction, and a food addict, just like any other addict, will do what is necessary to maintain the addiction and to keep others from challenging it or possibly eliminating it.

A food addict approaches their addiction like any other addict approaches theirs. They will do what they need to secure the food they want, while cost, health concerns, financial problems, physical problems, and collateral damage become nonessential points to consider. Family and physicians will warn them that their health is being compromised, and they will experience severe limitations in their mobility, motivation, and general health. When this happens, food becomes their drug of choice, and they become addicted to it, and they will protect their addiction at all costs.

THE STATISTICS - BULIMIA AND ANOREXIA

Here are recent statistics on bulimia and anorexia:[11]

➤ At any given time, 1% of young women and 0.1% of young men meet diagnostic criteria for bulimia nervosa, which makes it more common than anorexia nervosa(2-3 percent of women over their lifetime).

➤ The lifetime prevalence of bulimia in women is estimated between 1.2% to 4.6%.

➤ The median age of onset of bulimia and anorexia is eighteen years old.

➤ The lifetime prevalence for subthreshold bulimia in women by age twenty is 6.1%. "Subthreshold" refers to meeting all symptoms of bulimia, except one or more symptoms do not quite meet the diagnostic requirements. For example, bingeing or purging less than once a week on average.

➤ 95% of people with bulimia have at least one co-occurring mental health disorder. Between 36% and 50% of individuals with bulimia also have major depressive disorder, while between 54% and 81% are also diagnosed with anxiety disorder.

➤ High school students with disordered eating are more likely to use alcohol and other substances.

➤ Only 46% of people who have anorexia nervosa achieve full recovery, and 20% face lifelong health challenges and remain chronically ill due to the disorder.

➤ Up to 50% of people who have anorexia nervosa will develop bulimia nervosa over time.

➤ One in five people who pass away from anorexia nervosa die by suicide.

At the other end of the spectrum are the people who control every aspect of their food intake. They may understand that they need food to live, but they will control what goes in their mouth when they eat, how much they eat, and where they eat. The key focal points for these people are control, body image, self-esteem, and protection. They will eat smaller amounts of food and only certain foods at certain times. Some people will control food, but it will not progress to the point of nutritional problems or health issues. There may be control issues with food, but it does not necessarily progress to the point of addiction.

For some people with food control issues, they may continue to eat, but when they do, they feel an intense need to remove the food from their bodies. These people will eat, sometimes in large amounts, and then purge (vomit) their stomach contents. This eating disorder is known as bulimia and is characterized by uncontrolled episodes of overeating (called bingeing). This is followed by purging by self-induced vomiting, misuse of laxatives, and other methods. Bulimia typically affects females and usually starts during the teenage years. The characteristics of bulimia are:

➤ Usually a normal or above-average body weight

- Recurrent episodes of binge eating and fear of not being able to stop eating

- Self-induced vomiting (usually secretive)

- Excessive exercise

- Excessive fasting

- Peculiar eating habits or rituals

- Inappropriate use of laxatives or diuretics

For some people with food-control issues, as the condition progresses, they can become anorexic, and when this happens, all rational thought about food can be discarded. Anorexia, though it is not typically thought of as a food addiction, is an addiction designed to control food. For this type of addict, it is not the addiction to food that is the problem. It is the addiction to control it, and in its worst-case scenario, it can develop into avoidance of food altogether.

Just as a food addict who is protective of the food they love will do anything they can, even sacrifice their health to maintain their addiction, a person with anorexia will sacrifice everything to control their food intake, even if it threatens to end their life. When the addiction gets to this point, all rational perceptions are lost, and the addict cannot stop the process of avoiding food, protecting themselves, and arriving at a hypothetical body image that they may never achieve. Doctors and medical researchers do not know why people become anorexic. However, they know some conditions that make it more likely to occur. They can include:

- Being born female (females are more likely to be anorexic than males)

- Imbalance in neurotransmitter production

- Heredity and genetic disposition

- Higher childhood body mass index

- Social and family pressure to be thin

- Validation and abandonment issues

- Difficulty expressing feelings
- History of being teased about being fat
- History of sexual or physical abuse
- Perfectionism, or setting unrealistic standards
- A belief that a thinner body is ideal
- Unhappiness with body image
- Low self-esteem
- Depression, anxiety, stress, anger, or loneliness
- Excessive use of laxatives
- Excessive dieting
- A history of psychiatric disorders

In Chapter 8, I provided two progression sections, one for prescription-based amphetamines and the other for street-based amphetamines. I am going to follow the same design here as I present the progressions for food addiction and food control as it develops into bulimia and anorexia.

THE PROGRESSION—FOOD ADDICTION

1. The person may be dealing with issues stemming from abuse, neglect, and lack of safety, or they may have a genetic predisposition for addiction and have attached that to food.

2. The person begins with normal eating habits but with a stronger-than-normal enjoyment during the time they are eating.

3. The person begins to consume larger portions of food at meal times.

4. The person derives comfort from their eating experiences, and more food is consumed at mealtimes and between meals.

5. The user is beginning to identify foods that make them feel more comfortable.

6. As family members observe exaggerated eating habits, the user becomes defensive and refuses to discuss the matter.

7. The user begins to consume more food at meals and has begun hiding food and eating in secrecy.

8. The addict begins to hide stashes of food to be consumed when no one is watching them.

9. The addict continues to be defensive and is not paying attention to noticeable gains in weight.

10. Concerned about the opinions of others, the addict continues to eat larger portions at mealtimes and secretly delves into stashes.

11. The addict thinks about food excessively, plans their life around eating, and sets aside time for food, which has now become more important than other aspects of life.

12. The addict has fantasies about food and begins to establish eating rituals.

13. The addict has become protective about the food addiction, seems to be unconcerned about any form of collateral damage, and continues to carry out the eating rituals despite others' concerns.

14. Physical problems are developing, but the addict is unable to change their dysfunctional eating habits.

15. Experiencing physical problems, the addict visits the primary-care physician, who warns of the developing physical problems. The addict refuses to change the way they eat.

This is the typical progression that food addicts experience. Not all of them progress through the same steps and in the same way. For many, there is guilt, shame, and worry over what the addiction is doing to them, and many do want to stop the addiction and begin to eat more healthily. Unfortunately, without treatment, it is difficult for a food addict to stop the obsessive-compulsive behavior that drives the addiction. Since food must be consumed to survive, unlike other addictions, recovery can be difficult.

IN THE CLUTCHES

No addiction is free from the problems and side effects that develop from continued use. What follows is a list of the effects that one can experience from addiction to any drug or activity. Different addictions can lead to different problems, as you will see as we continue.

PHYSICAL PROBLEMS—The issues can include obesity, cardiovascular damage, high blood pressure, high cholesterol, structural damage, muscle damage, sleep apnea, gastrointestinal disorders, gastroesophageal reflux disease (GERD), and mobility issues.

MENTAL HEALTH ISSUES—Food addiction can cause severe self-image problems, depression, anxiety, obsessive-compulsive behaviors, shame, guilt, and isolation.

COMMUNICATION PROBLEMS—The only communication problems exist when the addict is avoiding other people and when they become defensive about the addiction. They often avoid communication because it may lead to discussions about their food addiction.

LEGAL PROBLEMS—There are no legal problems associated with food addiction.

FINANCIAL CONCERNS—Financial concerns are mild and usually associated with purchasing more food than is necessary.

FAMILY AND RELATIONSHIP ISSUES—Food addicts may avoid other family members to avoid confrontation, and in families where there is abuse, others may be verbally disrespectful toward the addict. Also, since the addict is defensive, they can become angry and mildly aggressive at times.

EMPLOYMENT PROBLEMS—There are generally no employment problems with food addicts unless their health begins to be a problem, which may interfere with their ability to maintain employment.

CHANGES IN SOCIAL LIFE—Any changes in social life are usually the result of an addiction that has progressed to the point that eating becomes more important than being with other people or because excessive weight gain or physical problems limit their mobility.

LYING—Food addicts will lie about how much they consume and how often. At times, their difficulty with honesty may spread into other areas of their lives, such as responsibilities, social life, and getting help for their addiction.

ACCOUNTABILITY ISSUES—Food addicts are typically accountable people. Still, there can be problems if the addiction progresses to the point that their consumption of food and their physical/mental health make it difficult for them to accept responsibility and follow through with responsibilities.

PERSONALITY CHANGES—Primary changes are a worsening of obsessive-compulsive behavior, rumination, and a tendency to rationalize and intellectualize their behaviors.

ANGER AND VIOLENCE—Typically, there are no appreciable differences in anger and violence. In some cases, food addicts can respond to others' remarks about their addiction with angry tones.

THE PROGRESSION—FOOD CONTROL BULIMIA AND ANOREXIA

"While bulimia nervosa is not technically classified as a type of addiction, many aspects of the disorder fit this definition. Many experts acknowledge the similarities between bulimia nervosa and addiction. They believe they are more interconnected than has likely been formally recognized." https://bulimia.com/bulimia-mental-illness/addictive/

There are two paths that people who control food can follow. Some control food to gain a low-grade sense of control over their environment. They are not concerned about controlling other people but do not want to feel out of control. This is often seen with bulimics and in the very early stages of anorexia. In more severe cases, food control can progress to the state of advanced anorexia. I am going to present the following progression to explain how food control begins and how it progresses to a point where it consumes the addict.

1. The person begins to control food as a way to divert attention away from pain, abuse, neglect, and safety issues and also to gain control over at least one part of their life since so much of their life seems out of control.

2. This often begins at a younger age when a child is a difficult eater, will only eat certain foods, and tends to eat smaller portions.

3. When challenged to eat more and eat healthier, the child resists the advances from parents and significant others.

4. The child begins to eat only certain foods and refuses to try those being suggested by parents and other adults.

5. Other significant people in the child's life begin to adjust to their eating style and don't challenge it so long as they feel the child is getting the nutrition they need.

6. As the child progresses into adolescence and life circumstances become challenging, the control over food increases.

7. Adolescents may refuse to eat foods with certain textures and typically have difficulty with fruits and vegetables.

8. They will eat certain select types of food and may rotate them every few days, but they will generally refuse to eat anything but those foods.

9. Body image is beginning to become an issue. This is especially true for females.

10. Control over food becomes more pronounced in anxious and challenging situations, especially when life changes are being introduced.

11. As the difficulties with life changes continue, the need for food control becomes more important and, at times, can become more pronounced.

12. When challenged about eating new foods, the person is more adamant than ever, has intellectualized their behavior, and has no attention whatsoever to change what they are doing.

For some people, control over food progresses to this point, and they either remain this way throughout their lives or make subtle changes as new and safer people and environments enter their lives, such as a safe and trusted relationship partner. For others, food control develops into a chronic and dysfunctional way of life. The person now begins to focus on issues beyond simple control.

1. Past issues of physical and sexual abuse, being harassed as a child, validation issues, trying to be perfect, body image issues, depression, anxiety, and loneliness create an atmosphere that is self-deprecating, shameful, and ridden with guilt.

2. Unlike their food-addict counterparts, food becomes the enemy and stands in the way of the control needed to survive.

3. Body image is everything, and the need for perfection establishes an inability to be satisfied with one's body, even when health becomes a serious issue.

4. This is where people become paranoid, untrusting, and unwilling to accept advice or assistance from anyone else.

5. Some will continue to eat in front of other people, but the feeling of food in their stomachs, and in particular, feeling full, causes them severe distress.

6. They may begin to purge (bulimia) immediately following meals to rid their body of the food they believe is toxic to them. This gives the semblance of eating to other people but allows the person to rid themselves of something they are having growing difficulty keeping inside them. For some, the eating disorder only progresses as far as bulimia.

7. Others are now focusing on weight issues and are becoming reluctant to consume even small amounts of food.

8. The obsessive-compulsive disorder is now substantial, and the person may firmly believe that consuming food could severely harm them.

9. The reduction of nutrients continues exacerbating the symptoms, but the person remains fixated on their body image.

10. Exercise and excessive use of laxatives are included in the plan.

11. The person is becoming argumentative, aggressive, and hostile. As with so many other addictions, they will do whatever they need to protect themselves and their plan.

12. Physicians are now warning that if the addict continues not eating, they will be hospitalized or, even worse, may lose their life.

13. The anorexic continues with the plan.

14. There is an emergency visit to the hospital, where conditions like cardiovascular and other organ damage are diagnosed, and the person may be placed in an inpatient program.

15. Sometimes, the person responds to treatment and begins a recovery program.

16. In other cases, they continue to refuse treatment, and they may lose their life.

IN THE CLUTCHES

PHYSICAL PROBLEMS (BULIMIA): Swelling around the cheeks and jaw, indigestion, frequent constipation, diarrhea, or new food intolerances. Heart-related conditions: irregular heartbeat and low blood pressure. Fainting or dizziness that is not due to another illness or health condition.

PHYSICAL PROBLEMS (ANOREXIA)—In the beginning stages, there are mood swings or changes in personality or judgment: difficulty speaking, slurred speech, or forgetting words; weakness; feeling dizzy or disorientated; an inability to concentrate; memory loss: headache and difficulty walking/problems with coordination. Later stages: cardiac or respiratory arrest; choking; suffocation, or strangulation; drug overdose; blood loss causing the blood pressure to drop; irregular heartbeat or damaged heart muscles being unable to pump enough blood and oxygen to the brain; other cardiovascular events, including heart attack, stroke, or heart failure; an acute asthma attack; inadequate oxygen supply or cardiac arrest while under general anesthesia; pneumonia; low hemoglobin levels in the blood; and sickle cell anemia or thalassemia.

MENTAL HEALTH ISSUES (BULIMIA)—There is sensitivity to comments about eating, dieting, exercise, or body image; feelings of shame, guilt, and disgust, especially after eating and/or purging; a distorted body image or extreme dissatisfaction with body shape; and anxiety or irritability around mealtimes.

MENTAL HEALTH ISSUES (ANOREXIA)—There is irritability, social withdrawal, lack of mood or emotion, inability to understand the seriousness of the situation, fear of eating in public, obsessions with food and exercise, depression, anxiety, paranoia, hallucinations, and suicidal ideation.

COMMUNICATION PROBLEMS—People suffering from bulimia and anorexia often appear to have a history of difficulty with both recognizing and communicating their need for emotional support and any emotional pain they are feeling. They have a difficult time discussing the trauma and pain that may have led to their addiction and any possible treatment to address these problems.

LEGAL PROBLEMS—There are few legal problems with bulimia or anorexia.

FINANCIAL CONCERNS—The problems associated with bulimia and anorexia have more to do with program and medical/counseling/psychiatric costs.

FAMILY AND RELATIONSHIP ISSUES—Bulimia and anorexia can cause many problems for family members. The conditions often result in a bulimic or anorexic person detaching from family members, and at times, they are often non-communicative. There is excessive worry on the part of family members, and many of them become anxious and depressed as a result of the pressure the condition causes. There may be repeated medical and hospital visits, psychiatric admissions, and, in severe cases, suicide attempts.

EMPLOYMENT PROBLEMS—There are no employment problems associated with bulimia In the early stages of anorexia, people tend to maintain employment; however, as the condition progresses, they develop physical problems to the point that they can no longer address the rigors of employment.

CHANGES IN SOCIAL LIFE—There are no severe social problems associated with bulimia. However, bulimics need to hide their purging, and this can lead to questions from friends and some distancing by the bulimic. Since anorexics tend to isolate from other people as the condition continues, there can be an extreme reduction in time spent in social situations.

LYING—Anorexics and bulimics will lie about their food intake, purging, and anything to do with food. They will do everything they can to protect themselves from others attempting to force food upon them.

ACCOUNTABILITY ISSUES—Bulimics who don't have other mental health concerns tend to maintain accountability concerning their responsibilities. In the early stages, anorexics typically can be counted upon to accept responsibility and complete tasks. However, considering the physical, mental, and emotional issues that develop as the condition continues, it is difficult to count on them to be responsible enough to handle their responsibilities.

PERSONALITY CHANGES—Bulimics can become more sensitive and express dissatisfaction with their life and the conditions that surround it. Anorexics can become isolated, protective, and almost antisocial. They are preoccupied with their body image, fearing what is happening in their life, and are always on guard to ensure others cannot sabotage their plans.

ANGER AND VIOLENCE—There seems to be no increase in anger or violence as bulimia progresses. The only time anger or violence develops is in the later stages of the condition when others are trying to make them eat more and eat healthier. They may react by becoming aggressive and violent. Anorexics, however, can become temperamental and angry as the condition progresses. At times, they can become violent.

Eating disorders such as bulimia tend to be caused by both physical and emotional problems. Treatment usually aims to address all these problems by reducing or eliminating binge eating and purging, treating physical complications caused by bulimia, helping the individual understand and change the emotional issues related to bulimia, identifying and treating any associated mental health disorders such as depression or anxiety, and encouraging and developing family support.

To help achieve these goals, nutritional counseling helps the individual develop a structured meal plan and understand and work with their purging triggers. Cognitive behavior therapy can help people with bulimia improve their body image, deal with their emotions, and create healthy eating behaviors. The plan might also include family and group psychotherapy as a positive support measure. Medications such as antidepressants may also be prescribed to help reduce the urge to binge and purge.

Identifying anorexia can be challenging. Secrecy, shame, and denial are characteristics of the disorder. As a result, the illness can go undetected for a long time. Although there are no lab tests to diagnose anorexia specifically, the doctor might use blood or urine tests to rule out physical illness as the cause of the weight loss. They also can look at how the person's organs are functioning. Imaging tests can check bone density. A cardiogram may be used to check the heart. The doctor may also refer the patient to a psychiatrist or a psychologist to address any mental or emotional concerns contributing to the condition.

To help treat anorexia, professionals use psychotherapy, medication if appropriate, nutritional counseling, group and family counseling, support groups, and follow-up medical care when necessary. In more severe cases, hospitalization may be part of the plan.

COLLATERAL DAMAGE

Food addictions, especially bulimia and anorexia, can take quite a toll on family dynamics. In the case of classic food addiction, where a person is addicted to eating food, the family's primary concerns revolve around the person's health. Even though there can be some communication issues and lying on the part of the food addict, the primary focus is usually on health. At times, communication issues can develop as the food addict becomes defensive about repeated attempts by others to help them with their addiction. For those who have addictions to eating and consume large amounts of food, weight gain and the corresponding physical problems can be severe.

In the cases of bulimia and anorexia, the effects on family dynamics can change drastically. Both of these can have significant impacts on a person's health, and there tend to be more mental health and emotional concerns associated with the conditions. The physical effects are more drastic, and as the addict's personality changes, there is always the possibility of anger and violence. In more severe cases, especially with anorexia, suicidal ideation can develop. In each case, past traumas and abuse could be part of the problem, and body image is typically part of both conditions.

Family members can be put through tremendous emotional pain watching their addicted family members suffer through their addictions. It is not uncommon for family members to seek counseling and other support measures to help them not only to address the problems the addict is experiencing but also to stay emotionally grounded. Some of the effects on family and significant others are intense and lead to emotional pain, insomnia, headaches, anxiety, depression, obsessive thoughts and worries, and medication to address some of these issues, such as antidepressants and antianxiety medications.

SUMMING IT UP

So often, food addictions and eating disorders are the result of past trauma and unresolved pain. If you believe that this may pertain to you, it is so important that you get help. Professional counselors are available to help you, and there are support groups who understand what you are experiencing and know what to do to help you. Try not to let past concerns and emotional issues dictate your physical and mental health. You are worth all the time it takes to get past this difficult condition. Be willing to get the help.

No addiction occurs in a void. Watching a family member slowly begin to lose their life is a harrowing way to live. Family members often feel helpless as they watch the life drain from another family member. Whether it is the classic food addiction, bulimia, or anorexia, each of them can leave family members horrified as they can only watch the conditions progress. The best advice for family members is to seek help from professionals who understand these conditions. Watching and doing nothing will leave you feeling trapped and helpless. The advice is the same as with any other addiction. Don't hide it, and don't enable the addiction. Talk about it and let others help you.

Food addicts can be resistant to treatment since food is a necessary part of their lives, and often, people don't consider food something that they may become addicted to. Also, in cases of bulimia and anorexia, since food is being avoided or purged, it is difficult to consider it an addiction. The addiction, in this case, is not so much about the food. It is about the process of avoiding food. That's what the person gets addicted to. The never-ending cycle of purging or avoiding food can progress to the point that one is left out of control, and this process may drastically affect their lives or, in some cases, end them. Every addiction has underlying obsessive-compulsive traits, and food-related addictions are no exception. Like any drug, left untreated, the results could be disastrous. If you are suffering from a food addiction or eating disorder, help is available for you.

Call the National Association of Anorexia Nervosa and Associated Disorders at 1 (888) 375-7767. Everything is confidential.

⏱ TIME TO TAKE ACTION

1. If you are addicted to food and cannot stop consuming it, there may be emotional reasons at the bottom of your addiction; start with your primary care physician and make an appointment with a counselor who understands food addictions.

2. For family members, as is the case with any addiction, talk to the professionals and learn as much as you can about what your family member is experiencing. Avoid trying to make a food addict eat less, a bulimic to stop purging, or an anorexic to start eating. Though all of these things may need to happen, for that to occur, they must understand the root causes of the addiction and obtain treatment to help address the causes of the problem.

3. In any addiction related to food, it is important to focus on the underlying motivation that causes the addiction. This could be physical, mental, emotional, or other underlying circumstances. Psychiatrists and psychologists with an expertise in food addictions can help you address these issues. Make an appointment with one.

4. If you don't know how to obtain counseling for a food addiction, start with your primary-care physician. They usually have people in their network who can address this condition.

5. Stay away from trying to make a food addict eat less, a bulimic to stop purging, or an anorexic to start eating. Though all of these things may need to happen, for that to occur, they must understand the root causes of the addiction and obtain treatment to help address the causes of the problem.

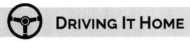

DRIVING IT HOME

Food addictions can be one of the more difficult addictions to treat. These addicts are often resistant, feel out of control, are distrustful of other people, and firmly believe that what they are doing is the right way to address what they are feeling. If you are addicted to food or are doing your best to either control your intake, purge what you are eating, or attempt to eat as little as possible, it can be a slippery slope, leading to horrible pain and potentially life-threatening problems. Eventually, the addiction catches up with you, and you will pay the price. Help is available if you are willing to accept it. For family members, the best way to help someone with a food addiction is to understand it and get help for it. Don't try to do this on your own. Start with your primary care physician.

YOUR DECLARATION IS: *I will come to terms with my food addiction, and I will get the help that can save my life!*

ONWARD

In the next chapter, I will examine the adrenaline rush that often accompanies gambling. Instead of discussing the chase to win the pot of gold, I will discuss the intense euphoric state that develops during active gambling. I will look at changes in a person's thinking, how it affects them emotionally, and the physical demands on their bodies as a result of acute and chronic gambling.

CHAPTER 12

◇◇◇◇◇◇◇◇◇◇◇◇◇

Gambling—
The Rush to Destruction

Winning has nothing to do with it. It's all about the rush . . .
a high-stakes straight line to disaster.

PROCESSES TO EMPLOY: Brutal Honesty, I Over E, Present-
Understand-Fix, Slowing Down Life's Pace, Internal Focus, Fact-
Finding, Honesty, Patience, Truth-Telling, Belief, Listening, Trust

---

GAMBLING IS WAGERING SOMETHING OF VALUE, USUALLY your
money, on a random event, intending to win something else of more
value. Gambling comes in many different forms. Commercial gambling
includes lotteries, instant lotteries, number games (such as Lotto and
Keno), sports betting, horse and dog race betting, poker and other card
games, casino table games (such as roulette and craps), bingo, and electronic gaming machines (EGMs). There are also illegal forms of gambling, such as high-stakes poker games, where the potential winnings are
considerably larger, as is the risk involved.

There are three common types of gamblers: the social gambler, the
professional gambler, and the problem gambler.

➤ **THE SOCIAL GAMBLER**—Social gamblers enjoy gambling occasionally. They are typically not high-stakes bettors. They may regularly
engage in monthly poker games with friends and occasionally visit
casinos. They typically have limits on how much they are willing to
spend, and for the most part, they gamble within those limitations.

➤ **THE PROFESSIONAL GAMBLER**—Professional gamblers gamble regularly for their primary income. Their proceeds are usually considered regular earned income and are taxed at normal income tax rates. They often set limits regarding the time spent gambling and have financial limits regarding how much will be spent at any given time.

➤ **THE ADDICTIVE GAMBLER**—Addictive gambling is the uncontrollable urge to gamble despite negative consequences in the gambler's life.

The type of gambling considered the most addictive has traditionally been slot machines. However, with the rise of Internet gambling sites, online gaming has become a top contender. The list of the different types of gambling is a long one, with the most prominent being:

➤ Sports betting

➤ Casino

➤ Bingo

➤ Lotteries

➤ Card games

➤ Poker

➤ Slot machines

➤ Baccarat

➤ Blackjack

➤ Craps

➤ Horse racing

➤ Roulette

➤ Gambling machines

➤ Raffles

➤ Scratch cards

➤ Betting pool

➤ British gambling games

➤ Dice

➤ Spinning wheels

At one time, gambling was illegal in most U.S. states. In the past decade, however, gambling has been legalized in most states across the nation, evolving to the point that one can access gambling apps on one's computer or smartphone. Gambling can be done right from one's home, twenty-four hours a day.

Compulsive gambling, also called gambling disorder, is the uncontrollable urge to keep gambling despite the toll it takes on one's life. Gambling can stimulate the brain's reward system, much like drugs or alcohol can, leading to addiction. Compulsive gambling may lead to the gambler continually chasing bets that lead to losses, using up savings, and creating debt. The addict may hide their behavior from others and even turn to theft or fraud to support their addiction.

THE STATISTICS

Here are recent statistics on gambling:[12]

➤ Up to 20 million Americans have or are at risk for gambling problems.

➤ Oklahoma has the highest rate of gambling addiction of all U.S. states, with 6.2% of their population addicted to gambling.

➤ The social cost for a gambling addict is over $30,000 per year.

➤ The prevalence of gambling addiction in men is one and one-half to two times more common than among women.

➤ 50.2% of all slot machine players have gambling problems.

➤ In 2022, U.S. players gambled for $250 billion, or $764 per capita.

➤ Slot machines are the most addictive; 75% of problem gamblers play slots.

➤ 81% of gambling addicts play online.

➤ 3% of American problem gamblers have more than $300,000 in gambling debts.

➤ Suicide rates among problem gamblers are fifteen times higher than that of the general population.

➤ 60% of problem gamblers smoke, and 26% are alcoholics.

THE PROGRESSION

1. A person usually starts gambling by making small bets, often with friends. They may limit their gambling to sports pools, a weekly lottery, or an occasional trip to the casino.

2. Others will enjoy the thrill of the bet and are focused on winning the wager.

3. The thrill associated with gambling increases adrenaline production and has a euphoric effect on neurotransmitters in the brain. These people will continue to gamble for the high it produces.

4. As the user's brains adjust to the euphoria and/or excitement gambling can produce, they continue to seek out gambling-related events. As with any addiction, as the tolerance builds, the gambler seeks a greater risk to continue to spike their excitement.

5. As the addiction develops, the users may increase lottery ticket purchases, increase their involvement in online betting, or make more trips to the casino.

6. Though the users set limits on how much they are willing to spend, those limits are often surpassed.

7. As the users gamble more often, their brains continue to adjust to the increases in neurotransmitter production gambling creates, and they begin to indulge in the behavior more often.

8. When this happens, gambling becomes a routine part of their lives. Still staying within reasonable financial limits, the time spent gambling and the amount of money begin to increase.

9. As the addiction takes hold, the addict is putting money away for gambling purposes.

10. Now, the addict will gamble as much as possible, not so much to win, but for the rush that occurs during the gambling experience.

11. As the addiction progresses, the addict is envisioning the big payday that most of them know may never occur. The environment where gambling occurs and the process of gambling produces the euphoria, and the action that surrounds the gambling process powers the addiction.

12. Some gambling addicts will begin to live paycheck to paycheck, always putting aside enough money to indulge in their addiction.

They will do their best not to put themselves in financial distress. Others will quickly blow past the limits and find themselves in debt, with their credit cards maxed out and bills unpaid. Unable to stop, they may begin to use investments and, at times, will be pushed to the point of bankruptcy.

13. For many addicts, this does not stop the gambling, and they will adjust their quality of life to accommodate the addiction.

WHY GAMBLE?

Some of the reasons people gamble are:

➤ For social reasons—This may be because it's what a group of friends do when they get together or because it makes a social gathering more enjoyable.

➤ For financial reasons—To win money because they enjoy thinking about what they would do if they won a jackpot or because winning would change their lifestyle.

➤ For entertainment reasons—They like the rush, or "high," because it makes them feel good.

➤ For coping reasons—To forget their worries, to feel more self-confident, or because it helps when they are feeling nervous or depressed.

Gambling can be an escape for people who have experienced a stressful change in life, such as relationship issues or money troubles. Others may start gambling because they are lonely and crave company. For many people, gambling is an addictive drug. Gambling disorders have been linked to variations in a variety of brain regions, particularly the striatum and prefrontal cortex, which are involved in reward processing, social and emotional problems, and stress. When these areas of the brain are stimulated, and as the brain continually adjusts to a higher level of excitement, it does its best to repeat the higher level of neurological gratification. It wants more and more of a good thing.

The excitement produced in the gambling environment excites those centers of the brain. Though the gambling addict is focusing on the game, it is the high-intensity immediate gratification that is at the root of the addiction. Like any other drug, when the person is not using (not gambling), there is a sharp reduction in the neurological stimulation to which the brain has adjusted and does its best to repeat. When this stimulation is not occurring, the user will experience withdrawal effects similar to any other drug addiction.

IN THE CLUTCHES

No addiction is free from the problems and side effects that develop from continued use. What follows is a list of the effects that one can experience from addiction to any drug or activity. Different addictions can lead to different problems, as you will see as we continue.

PHYSICAL PROBLEMS—From a medical perspective, pathological gamblers are at increased risk of developing stress-related conditions, such as hypertension, sleep deprivation, cardiovascular disease, and peptic ulcer disease.

MENTAL HEALTH ISSUES—Mental health effects include exacerbation and initiation of major depressive episodes, anxiety disorders, or substance use disorders. Psychological consequences may also include intense levels of guilt and shame, deceptive practices, heightened impulsivity, and impaired decision-making.

COMMUNICATION PROBLEMS—The communication between gamblers and those close to them often becomes aggressive, argumentative, and evasive as the gamblers do their best to continue with the excitement the addiction provides while, at the same time, stopping others from interfering with their addiction.

LEGAL PROBLEMS—Legal problems associated with gambling can come from the aggressive behavior resulting from drinking and drug abuse while gambling, involvement in illegal gambling enterprises, sports betting, especially by athletes, and aggressive behavior that can result during and after a gambling event. White-collar crimes like fraud, theft, and embezzlement often occur in cases of severe debt.

FINANCIAL CONCERNS—The financial problems associated with gambling can range from minor inconveniences to all-encompassing debt. Some gamblers will lose a safe, self-designated amount during each gambling event. In contrast, others routinely exceed their limits, face severe financial problems, and can lose their homes and enter bankruptcy.

FAMILY AND RELATIONSHIP ISSUES—Like any addiction, gambling can consume the addict. Large amounts of time are spent away from family members and family-related events. Excessive amounts of money are spent, leading to arguments and, in many cases, separations and divorces. Money is not available for the needs of the family, and often, substance abuse exacerbates an already difficult problem. Family members can grow intolerant to the addiction and the uncaring attitude of the addict. They understand that if the addiction continues, they may lose everything. They may decide to sever the relationship with the gambling addict to protect themselves.

EMPLOYMENT PROBLEMS—Gambling usually doesn't cause problems with employment unless the person progresses to the point where they spend significant amounts of time in poker games, online, and at the casino. When gambling progresses to this point, like many other addictions, it becomes the priority in one's life, and employment can suffer. In severe cases, people will miss work to attend gambling events. Problem gambling can result in disciplinary actions and, at times, termination,

CHANGES IN SOCIAL LIFE—The social consequences of addictive gambling can be enormous since the addict can become unconcerned about spending time with other people unless those times are connected to gambling.

LYING—Gamblers will lie about how often they are gambling, how much time they spend with this addiction, and how much money they are spending. They will often lie about their winnings and any other information that may support their addiction. They will lie about their finances and say anything they need to support the addiction.

ACCOUNTABILITY ISSUES—Accountability suffers as the addiction progresses. In cases where substance abuse is part of the problem, there can be low levels of commitment and accountability. Gamblers will often deprioritize family and home-related responsibilities as they continue to dedicate more time to the addiction.

PERSONALITY CHANGES—Gambling is a fast, intense addiction. The personality changes addicts experience include substance abuse problems, personality disorders, depression, or anxiety. There are also increases in obsessive-compulsive thoughts and behaviors.

ANGER AND VIOLENCE—The intensity that comes with a gambling addiction often translates into angry and volatile behaviors. The adrenaline rush is at its height during the active gambling phase but also proceeds well into times when the addict is not gambling. They can also become angry and violent during periods of withdrawal from the addiction. Confrontations with other gamblers, casino security, friends, law-enforcement personnel, and family members can, at times, accelerate into violent episodes.

Like so many other addictions, gambling is a destructive, progressive disorder. As opposed to focusing on winning, which often occurs in the early stages and with social gamblers, when gambling progresses to the point of addiction, it can change almost every aspect of one's life. The legalization of gambling has further exacerbated the problem, and the advent of online gambling has made it accessible virtually anytime.

When gambling progresses to the point of addiction, it is no longer about winning and losing. There is no pot of gold at the end of the rainbow; addicted gamblers typically understand this, though they may not admit it. Though they all talk about the big payday, the truth is that it's about the ride, the adrenaline rush, and the euphoria that comes from being in the game. When gambling progresses to this point, almost everything else in an addict's life takes a back seat. When this happens, it doesn't take long for a gambling addict to lose most of what they have.

COLLATERAL DAMAGE

The collateral damage that happens at the hands of a gambling addict touches almost every aspect of family life. For a family whose finances were stable and who had money in the bank for those rainy days, gambling can drain the family's accounts and cause considerable financial damage. Emotionally, family members experience anxiety, depression, and physical ailments such as abdominal problems, headaches, and excessive worrying. Family members find themselves ruminating over what may occur if the problem continues, and when it does get to the point of crisis, they must find a way to survive the damage the gambling addict has done. This may include leaving the addict.

Even in the most loving households, gambling, lying, substance abuse, long hours away from the family, financial distress, and obsessive-compulsive behaviors can turn a home that is loving and supportive into one that is angry and, at times, violent. In addition, gamblers can amass huge debts and find themselves in the position of, at the very least, needing to pay credit-card balances with huge interest rates and, at worst, involving themselves with loan sharks and other potentially violent financial enterprises.

Family members are at risk not only of experiencing all the problems that gambling causes within the family, but they might also be at risk of being placed in dangerous situations, such as entanglements with loan sharks and bookmakers, as the gambling addict does whatever they can to stay involved in the game.

SUMMING IT UP

Gambling is an addiction that can consume an individual, destroy their family relationships, and wreck their finances. It has become one of the leading addictions as it is attached to sports betting and casino access on the Internet. Without leaving the comforts of one's home, one can access online betting programs and indulge in an activity that can monopolize them and change the scope of their entire life.

For some, gambling exists in close connection with other addictions, like drug and alcohol abuse. It is not uncommon for bills to go unpaid, credit cards to be maxed out, and family savings to be exhausted, and for some, their lives will end in bankruptcy. Like any other entertainment activity, when performed responsibly and only occasionally, gambling can be an innocent and enjoyable addition to life. Setting spending limits and never exceeding those limits is the healthy formula to enjoy gambling but not have it take control of your life.

For some people, however, gambling becomes an addiction, and that addiction can destroy their identity and everyone they touch. If you feel as though gambling is an addiction in your life, don't wait. The exhilaration you feel at the hands of this addiction is only temporary, but the damage can be permanent.

Help is available through the National Problem Gambling Helpline: call 1 (800) GAMBLER or text 800GAM.

 ### TIME TO TAKE ACTION

1. If you know you have a gambling problem, you can get help by working with an addictions counselor or by contacting the National Council on Problem Gambling.

2. You can also contact Gamblers Anonymous at (909) 931-9056 or search online to find out where they meet in your area. Attend your first meeting.

3. If you are a family member of a gambler, don't keep the problem to yourself. Make an appointment with a counselor who can connect you with support people to help you work through the problems the gambler's addiction is causing in your life.

4. Make an appointment with your primary care physician to address any physical issues that may be developing from the stress that comes with gambling addictions.

5. Gambling has become a serious financial problem, and whether you are the gambler or the family member, contact your accountant or a financial consultant who can help you address the financial concerns that may be developing or have developed.

6. For family members, make an appointment with an attorney to protect your rights should the gambling progress to the point that it threatens your economic welfare.

DRIVING IT HOME

Compulsive gambling is a serious condition that can destroy lives. Although treating it can be challenging, many people who struggle with this addiction have found help through professional treatment. Support for this problem is available through counseling services, gambling support groups, psychiatrists who can help in cases where medication is necessary, and family support programs to help repair the collateral damage.

YOUR DECLARATION IS: *I will get help for my gambling addiction, and I will learn to live without this life-destroying addiction!*

ONWARD

In the next chapter, I will look at the addiction to smartphones, video games, and other electronics. I will examine how addiction to these devices can carry the same neurological addictive processes as drug abuse.

CHAPTER 13

Smartphones and Video Games— Machine Mind Control

It is the most insidious surrender of the human will and has become the most socially prevalent addiction in history.

PROCESSES TO EMPLOY: Brutal Honesty, I Over E, Present-Understand-Fix, Slowing Down Life's Pace, Internal Focus, Fact-Finding, Honesty, Patience, Truth-Telling, Belief, Listening, Trust

---

IN TODAY'S FAST-PACED ELECTRONIC AGE, ALMOST EVERYONE owns or has access to a smartphone or a computer. Smartphone addiction may be categorized as a behavioral addiction that presents when a person can't go without their smartphone, when their excessive use causes adverse consequences, or when they experience symptoms similar to withdrawal when they aren't using their device. Today's smartphones aren't only used for making phone calls. A tremendous amount of time is spent on these devices, engaging in social media postings and videos. Today's smartphones are actually computers with a cell phone component built into them.

While addiction to one's smartphone may be a reality for many, it is not officially recognized as a mental health illness or an addiction in the fifth edition of the *Diagnostic and Statistical Manual of Mental Health Disorders* (DSM-5). However, it does present with similar characteristics to other behavioral addictions, such as drug addiction and gambling.

The exact number of people addicted to their smartphones isn't known. This is because it can be hard to quantify, and many studies base their data on self-reporting methods. People may not understand how to report their use accurately, and people aren't always truthful when self-reporting.

Although anyone can be at risk for this type of addiction, it is typically thought of as an enterprise for younger people. However, adults often demonstrate the same obsessive behaviors as their younger counterparts. People who get smartphones, iPads, and tablets at a younger age are also more likely to present with addictive behaviors than those who get them later in life.

Phone addiction may lead to:

➤ Lower concentration

➤ Aggravated ADD and ADHD

➤ Family and relationship problems

➤ Anxiety

➤ Reduced cognitive processing

➤ Reduced face-to-face socialization

➤ Stress

➤ Sleep deficits

➤ Poor study habits and lower grades

➤ Increased potential for employment problems

Video game addiction, also called Internet gaming disorder, as I am discussing it, is a condition characterized by severely reduced control over gaming habits. This condition can negatively affect many aspects of one's life, including communication, self-care, relationships, school, and work. This condition can include gaming on the Internet or any electronic device. Most people who develop significant gaming issues primarily play on the Internet.

Video game addiction can affect children, teens, and adults, although adults are most likely to have this condition. Males are thought of as more likely to become addicted to Internet gaming than females, but the number of females showing addictive tendencies to gaming seems to be increasing.

Signs and symptoms of video game addiction include:

➤ Poor performance at school, work, or household responsibilities due to excessive video game playing.

➤ Withdrawal symptoms, such as sadness, anxiety, or irritability, when games are taken away or gaming isn't possible.

➤ A need to spend more and more time playing video games to get the same level of enjoyment.

➤ Giving up other previously enjoyed activities or social relationships due to gaming.

➤ Being unable to reduce playing time or quit gaming despite the negative consequences it is causing.

➤ Lying to family members or others about the time spent playing video games.

➤ A decline in personal hygiene or grooming due to excessive video gaming.

➤ Using video games to escape stressful situations at work or school or avoid conflicts at home.

➤ Using video games to provide a distraction from past traumas and negative feelings, such as guilt or hopelessness.

Although there is no current diagnosis for smartphone addiction, the American Psychiatric Association (APA) included Internet gaming disorder (IGD) in the appendix of the DSM-5 as a potential diagnosis. Referring to the diagnostic criteria for substance use disorders, the DSM-5 drafted diagnostic criteria for IGD and indicated that further research is warranted. The requirements (paraphrased) are:

- Withdrawal symptoms when gaming is taken away or not possible (sadness, anxiety, irritability)

- Tolerance, the need to spend more time gaming to satisfy the urge

- Inability to reduce playing, unsuccessful attempts to quit gaming

- Giving up other activities, loss of interest in previously enjoyed activities due to gaming

- Continuing to game despite problems

- Deceiving family members or others about the amount of time spent on gaming

- The use of gaming to relieve negative moods, such as guilt or hopelessness

- Risk, having jeopardized or lost a job or relationship due to gaming use disorders

THE STATISTICS

Here are recent statistics on smartphone and video game addiction:[13]

Smartphones

1. The average American checks their phones 144 times per day.

2. 89% of Americans say they check their phones within 10 minutes of waking up.

3. 75% of Americans feel uneasy leaving their phone at home.

4. 75% of Americans check their phones within five minutes of receiving a notification.

5. 75% use their phone on the toilet.

6. 69% have texted someone in the same room as them before.

7. 60% sleep with their phone at night.

8. 57% consider themselves "addicted" to their phones.

9. 55% say they have never gone longer than 24 hours without their phone.

10. 47% of people say they feel a sense of panic or anxiety when their phone battery goes below 20%.

11. 46% use or look at their phone while on a date.

12. 27% use or look at their phone while driving.

Video Games

1. By the end of 2022, more than 2 billion people played video games worldwide, reaching 3 billion by 2023.

2. In the United States, 3% to 4% of gamers are addicted to video games. As many as 60 million people (or more) suffer from gaming disorder.

3. In the United States, between 0.3% and 1% of the general population have symptoms associated with gaming disorder.

4. 8.5% of youths aged between 8 and 18 suffer from gaming disorder.

5. 49% of all American adults have played video games, but only 10% consider themselves "gamers." [14]

Smartphone and Internet gaming addictions follow the same addictive patterns we see with alcohol and drug addiction. A tolerance for the activity is created, the mind adjusts to it, and obsession develops, followed by increased dependence and, finally, an addiction. Since electronic devices are virtually always available, it is difficult to separate oneself from them, especially with smartphones. Unlike landlines, smartphones go where the user goes. During one's waking hours, they are often connected to the person in some manner. Even when one is sleeping, they are right by their side, always on and ready for action.

Though we tend to view smartphone addiction as something experienced primarily by younger people, it is important to note that smartphones have been part of the culture for almost thirty years. Today, adults are just as likely to be addicted to smartphones as adolescents. Conversely, gaming tends to be something adults attach themselves to more often than children. Adolescents, being tech-savvy people, are very knowledgeable about the gaming industry and do show addictive tendencies to Internet gaming. These adolescents, maturing into adulthood, are at serious risk of continuing their addictive smartphone and other electronic addictions into adulthood.

THE PROGRESSION

Though once someone is in the grasp of smartphone and gaming addictions, the problems it creates are similar to alcohol and drug addiction, the progression of each addiction is a bit different. I will present the progressions from use to addiction separately; however, in the "In the Clutches" section, where I present the problems addicted users experience, they are much the same and will be presented together.

Smartphone Addiction

1. The person acquires a smartphone and uses it sporadically for phone calls, texting, and taking pictures.

2. The user begins adding people to their contact list, increasing texting and smartphone use.

3. Texting and phone calls continue throughout the day and begin to expand into later evening hours.

4. The user begins accessing the Internet via smartphone and browsing intermittently.

5. The user now texts throughout the day, spends more time on social media, and texts those on their contact list more often.

6. The user begins to rely on the smartphone to enhance their social life and stay connected with friends and social issues.

7. Smartphone use begins to interfere with other parts of life as the smartphone begins to define life socially and personally.

8. The addict is using the phone for large amounts of time during the day and often at inappropriate times, such as at work and during class.

9. The addict is neglecting responsibilities and distancing themselves from other people as smartphone use continues to increase.

10. The addict opens their day with smartphone use and often uses it long into the evening to the point that their sleep patterns are affected.

11. The addict is having a difficult time being without their phone. If they lose their phone, the battery dies, or they are placed in situations where smartphones may not apply or there is no service, they become uncomfortable and often angry.

12. The addict can no longer be without the smartphone, as it and their lives have become inseparable. Separation from the device can be terrifying.

Internet Gaming Addiction

1. The person acquires a computer and begins to use it for e-mail, work or school activities, and Internet surfing.

2. The person is exposed to and begins playing their first Internet game.

3. Liking the game, the person spends more time playing it.

4. The person discovers how to play online games with other players.

5. The person joins an Internet gaming group and begins playing games with others on the Internet at selected times.

6. The person may join gaming clubs, become more knowledgeable about the various Internet games and how to play them, and expand the amount of time spent playing them.

7. The user researches gaming computers and purchases a more powerful computer to enhance their gaming experience.

8. The user is now playing Internet games more and may have joined several Internet gaming groups.

9. The user is beginning to increase their skill level, spending considerably more time in the games, and responsibilities are beginning to be neglected.

10. The user is staying up late to play games, and their sleep schedules are becoming interrupted.

11. The addict is becoming consumed with Internet gaming, talks about it often, and continues purchasing new computers and components to enhance the gaming experience and become more efficient and competitive.

12. The addict is becoming more intense, at times, and more argumentative while playing, and both their sleep and dietary health are beginning to suffer.

13. When challenged about excessive game playing, the addict will become defensive and, at times, verbally abusive.

14. The addict begins to exhibit disregard for responsibilities and the feelings of others who are caught in their addiction.

15. The addict plays Internet games every day, often several times per day, and at times may play for the better part of the day and well into the evening.

16. The addict experiences periods of withdrawal, where they become intolerant and obsess about getting back to the game.

17. The addict has a difficult time living life without Internet gaming.

Consistent with any addiction, the progression from use through abuse and into addiction can be different for different people. However, as you may note in both progressions, though there are some differences, the main theme is the same: The person initially uses the smartphone or the Internet responsibly but progresses through abusive use and into addiction.

IN THE CLUTCHES

No addiction is free from the problems and side effects that develop from continued use. What follows is a list of the effects that one can experience from addiction to any drug or activity. Different addictions can lead to different problems, as you will see as we continue.

PHYSICAL PROBLEMS—Physical issues associated with Internet gaming disorder include headaches, body aches, nutritional issues, sleep deprivation, neurological over-acceleration, carpal tunnel syndrome, and increased physical stress.

MENTAL HEALTH ISSUES—Impulsivity, low self-control, anxiety, obsessive-compulsive problems, and lower positive affect are among the mental health problems associated with Internet gaming disorder.

COMMUNICATION PROBLEMS—Communication suffers as addicts begin to spend more time on their devices, isolate during usage, and substitute phones and games for interpersonal communication experiences.

LEGAL PROBLEMS—There are no increases in legal problems with either device; however, texting while driving has caused legal problems due to accidents and police checkpoints.

FINANCIAL CONCERNS—Financial concerns are primarily relegated to the high cost of purchasing smartphones and gaming equipment. Online purchases have increased, causing people to spend more time engaged in impulsive shopping.

FAMILY AND RELATIONSHIP ISSUES—Family and relationship issues develop because smartphone and Internet gaming involvement challenges family and interpersonal time. Texting has replaced personal communication for many people, and gaming absorbs a considerable amount of family time.

EMPLOYMENT PROBLEMS—The only employment-related issue seems to be the inappropriate use of smartphones and tablets during work hours.

CHANGES IN SOCIAL LIFE—The changes in social life are related to less time spent on personal communication and human contact. As opposed to personal contact, people spend more time involved in electronic contact, where social life can be defined by distant communication.

LYING—The only lying that seems to increase is the amount of time spent on smartphones and in gaming experiences.

ACCOUNTABILITY ISSUES—As usage increases, accountability tends to decrease. It is difficult to be accountable when one's priority is an electronic device that consumes so much time.

PERSONALITY CHANGES—Smartphone and gaming addicts often experience reductions in creativity, ambition, compassion, flexibility, conscientiousness, reliability, and agreeableness.

ANGER AND VIOLENCE—Any instances of anger or violence seemed to be connected to challenges by family members and significant others regarding the amount of time one spends engaged in smartphone and gaming activities. Most of these instances are verbal expressions of anger; however, smartphone and gaming addicts can become violent if their devices are taken from them or when they are in withdrawal from their selected devices.

COLLATERAL DAMAGE

Collateral damage as a result of both smartphone and Internet gaming addiction is initially seen as one begins to withdraw from family activities, communication, and responsibilities. Family members of the addicts must adjust to less communication and more irresponsible behavior as a result of enhanced usage.

Family members can experience the addict's anger and stubbornness should they challenge the addict about their usage time, personality changes, lack of responsibility, and changing attitude. Considerably less time is spent with other family members or in family activities. Those activities demand that less time is spent on the addiction, and smartphone and gaming addicts have a problem with that. Even when they may be involved in a family activity, they remain connected to their smartphone or the Internet.

SUMMING IT UP

Smartphones and Internet gaming are here to stay. They have become institutions across the globe, and almost everything humans do today is connected to smartphones and the Internet in some fashion. People firmly believe they need both and live much of their lives connected to these devices. They communicate with them, set their schedules, and run almost every aspect of their lives using smartphones, the Internet, or both.

Balance is always the key to healthy living. There is nothing wrong with texting other people routinely, surfing the Internet, or being involved in Internet gaming. The advice is to set time limits before becoming involved in these activities. If you cannot, it is a strong indication that you are addicted. Any addiction comes with consequences. If you are addicted to these devices, it makes good sense to get help. This increased level of use may be normalized in society, but that doesn't mean it's normal or, for that matter, healthy.

If you feel that you or someone close to you may be addicted to smartphones or other electronic devices, you can call the Addiction Center hotline at (870) 515-8609.

 TIME TO TAKE ACTION

1. Count how many calls and texts you make daily.

2. Keep track of how many hours you or any of your family members spend making smartphone calls, texting, or surfing the Internet.

3. To determine if you or any of your family members are addicted to your smartphone, turn it off and don't use it for one day. If it is

the only one you have for emergencies, do this in conjunction with another person who has a phone and can make emergency calls if necessary. Be honest and report how you feel when you disconnect from your electronics.

4. Keep track of how many hours you or your family members spend playing Internet games daily.

5. List all the purchases you or any of your family members have made to enhance your gaming experience. Now, rank those purchases with other household expenses.

6. To determine if you or any of your family members are addicted to Internet gaming, turn off the computer and don't use it for one day. Be honest and report how you feel about that.

7. If you are having difficulty disconnecting from your devices, it may be a sign that you have a smartphone and/or Internet gaming addiction. If you do, it's a good idea to get help for this. You can call a counselor or the number above to help you with your addiction.

 ## DRIVING IT HOME

Millions of people across the world play video games and Internet games. While the majority of people who enjoy these types of games do not develop problematic behaviors, it is possible for gaming to become all-consuming and negatively impact your daily functioning. If you are worried about your gaming habits or those of a loved one, contact your healthcare provider. They are always available to help you. Likewise, if you spend inordinate amounts of time on your smartphone, try to reduce that time and spend more time with family members or friends. If you cannot, consider getting help from a professional counselor.

YOUR DECLARATION IS: *I will reduce my involvement with electronics and spend more time with my family and friends!*

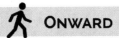

ONWARD

In the next chapter, I will discuss surrendering to the more primitive human drives as I look at power, control, secrecy, and fantasy. I will discuss how sex addictions can have a drastic effect on the way a person thinks and on their version of sexual reality.

CHAPTER 14

◇◇◇◇◇◇◇◇◇◇◇◇

Sex Addiction—
Exploitation Extraordinaire

It is a pitiful example of the human masterpiece stuck in a world of primal obsessions and empty fantasy.

PROCESSES TO EMPLOY: Brutal Honesty, I Over E, Present-Understand-Fix, Slowing Down Life's Pace, Internal Focus, Fact-Finding, Honesty, Patience, Truth-Telling, Belief, Listening, Trust

SEXUAL ADDICTION, TODAY REFERRED TO AS SEX ADDICTION, was first named and diagnosed in 1983 by Patrick Carnes, an internationally known authority and speaker on addiction and recovery issues. It is characterized by unrelenting obsessive thoughts and compulsive behaviors that often lie outside of normal sexual parameters. Compulsive sexual behavior is sometimes called hypersexuality or sexual addiction. It is an intense focus on sexual fantasies, urges, or behaviors that cannot be controlled.

Sexual addiction is a state that includes **compulsive** participation or engagement in sexual activity, such as:

➤ **PORNOGRAPHY**—The viewing of sexually explicit pictures and videos.

➤ **VOYEURISM**—Secretly viewing the actions of others who may be engaged in sexual activity.

➤ **PROSTITUTION**—The buying of another's body for sex or the selling of one's body for profit.

➤ **FANTASY**—Mental creations of sexually explicit and arousing situations.

➤ **MASTURBATION**—Manually manipulating the genitals to arrive at a climax. This is usually performed during periods of fantasy.

➤ **SADISTIC OR MASOCHISTIC BEHAVIOR**—Hurting oneself or others or allowing oneself to be hurt by others to attain the sexual climax.

➤ **EXHIBITIONISM**—Sexual gratification that is achieved through the indecent exposure of one's genitals, often to a stranger.

➤ **SEXUAL INTERCOURSE**—Sexual contact between individuals involving penetration.

In sexual addiction, the concern is the compulsive participation in these behaviors and the inability to stop oneself from continued involvement. This does not mean that engaging in these behaviors is dysfunctional. The concern, as with any other addiction, is the inability to stop, or at least reduce, the compulsion without experiencing the effects of withdrawal. Sex addicts will involve themselves in these behaviors as often as possible, regardless of any negative consequences that may develop.

The term "sexual dependence" is also used to refer to people who report being unable to control their sexual urges, behaviors, or thoughts. Related or synonymous models of pathological sexual behavior include hypersexuality (nymphomania and satyriasis), erotomania (excessive sexual desire), Don Juanism (the desire of a man to have sex with many female partners), and paraphilia-related disorders.

Like any other addiction, the defining measure of sexual addiction is the inability to stop the behavior. Sexual urges are a normal part of human thought and behavior and serve two important purposes:

1. Sexual activity, an innate human drive, increases the production of neurotransmitters, providing a healthy outlet for the brain.

2. Sexual activity leading to procreation furthers the continuation of the human species.

The sex drive is closely connected to the brain's pleasure center, and indulgence in sexual activity causes that center of the brain to experience euphoric pleasure.

THE STATISTICS

Here are recent statistics on sex and pornography addiction:[15]

1. 21 million Americans are sex addicts.

2. Two out of three sex addicts are men.

3. 93% of sex addicts also suffer from porn addiction.

4. One out of three men self-report that they feel addicted to porn.

5. 98% of sex addicts with a partner feel rejected by their partner.

6. Only 5% of addicts who go into rehab recover from the addiction.

7. 72% of sex addicts relapse in under six months after joining rehab.

8. 81% of sex addicts were sexually abused in childhood.

9. 72% of sex addicts were physically abused in childhood.

10. 97% of sex addicts were emotionally abused in childhood.

11. Three out of five sex addicts self-report posting naked photos of themselves online regularly.

12. On average, male sex addicts have had 32 sexual partners.

13. Female sex addicts report to have had 22 sexual partners on average.

14. 40% of sex addicts displayed symptoms of substance abuse.

15. 72% of sex addicts displayed symptoms of depression.

16. 23% of sex addicts displayed symptoms of bipolar disorder.

17. Children of households where parents displayed sexually addictive behavior are 22 times more likely to become sexually addicted later in life.

18. 37 new porn videos are made every day in the United States.

19. In the United States, 28,000 people are watching porn at any given moment.

20. About $3,000 is spent every second on pornographic material.

21. 35% of all downloads on the Internet are related to porn.

THE PROGRESSION

As with most addictions, sexual addiction follows a progression that applies to almost every type of addiction. However, in the case of voyeurs and exhibitionists, the progression to intercourse or physical contact with another person may not be necessary. In these cases, watching others or exposing themselves to others may be all that is needed to achieve arousal and, at times, climax.

Also, different people are exposed to sex at different times and in different ways. For some sex addicts, their childhood was void of any abuse or sexual trauma, and they did not experience any problems in adolescence. For others, they may have been abused as children, experienced some trauma during childhood or adolescence, or may have been exposed to alternative sexual expressions during childhood or adolescence. The progression for them could be accelerated and follow different guidelines.

Some people, as discussed in previous chapters, have an addictive personality, and their drug of choice is sex. If one is predisposed to addictive behaviors, their propensity for addictive thoughts and behavior may have engaged with sex as its centerpiece.

1. The individual is exposed to one of the types of sex listed earlier in the chapter.

2. Initially, the individual refrains from any form of sexual activity. This may be for religious or moral reasons, fear of others finding out, or stigmas regarding sex that are learned from family or significant others.

3. The individual has their first sexual experience. This could be with pornography or voyeurism.

4. The images of what the person saw leave a lasting physical, emotional, and/or intellectual impression. They excite the person, and they begin to look for similar experiences.

5. The person begins to engage in fantasy after additional viewing of sexual-related material or watching other people engage in sexual behavior that may range from simple kissing or petting to explicit sexual acts.

6. The person begins to think about sex even when no viewing material is available and begins to engage in sexual fantasies.

7. The person begins to touch themselves sexually during fantasies, followed by an initial experience with masturbation.

8. Understanding this as an easy way to achieve sexual gratification, the individual continues to fantasize and masturbate.

9. As the addiction progresses, and masturbation, though pleasurable, does not satisfy all sexual needs, the individual seeks out a sex partner.

10. The individual experiences sex with another person for the first time, feels the excitement and the euphoria, and now thinks about sex at varying times throughout the day.

11. Indulging in pornography increases, and the addict begins to watch videos depicting various forms of sexual behavior.

12. The addict begins to schedule times every day to engage in some form of sexual activity. This could be watching pornography, fantasy, masturbation, voyeurism, exhibitionism, or sex with another person.

13. When none of these vehicles are available, the addict can become restless, temperamental, and uncomfortable physically, emotionally, and intellectually.

14. The addiction is now something that must be satisfied as often as possible to keep the person happy and to avoid the unpleasant withdrawal that abstention produces.

It is important to note that this is the usual progression from the healthy sexual beginner to the sexual addict. In cases of abuse, rape, and other sexual trauma, individuals can progress through the stages differently and at a different pace. Some are introduced to the later stages of the progression quite early, and they may show signs of the addiction as early as childhood.

IN THE CLUTCHES

No addiction is free from the problems and side effects that develop from continued use. What follows is a list of the effects that one can experience from addiction to any drug or activity. Different addictions can lead to different problems, as you will see as we continue.

PHYSICAL PROBLEMS—Physical risks of sexual addiction include exposure to sexually transmitted diseases, genital harm from intense masturbation, and exposure to HIV and hepatitis B and C.

MENTAL HEALTH ISSUES—Feelings of betrayal, abandonment, humiliation, depression, isolation, loneliness, guilt, shame, and anger are among the mental health effects of sex addiction. Also, normal sexual activity is replaced by an obsessive compulsion regarding sexual thoughts and behaviors.

COMMUNICATION PROBLEMS—As the addiction progresses and feelings of guilt and shame grow, the amount and quality of communication with family, friends, and loved ones are often reduced. Should family members discover the addiction, they may become hurt or angry, and this could have a more serious impact on communication.

LEGAL PROBLEMS—Legal problems can result for voyeurs if they are discovered and in cases related to prostitution and exhibitionism. In some cases, charges may be filed against the addict, resulting in fines, probation, and, in more severe cases, incarceration.

FINANCIAL CONCERNS—Financial concerns can arise in cases related to prostitution and for court costs and fines that result from legal charges when laws related to sexual conduct are violated.

FAMILY AND RELATIONSHIP ISSUES—Family relationships can be affected as the sexual addict pulls away from family members to engage in their addiction and when family members discover the addiction and disapprove of what the addict is doing. Relationships can suffer significantly as other family members become angry, embarrassed, hurt, and rejected by the addict, who is actively involved in the addiction.

EMPLOYMENT PROBLEMS—Typically, there are no problems associated with employment. However, at times, individuals might watch pornography on company computers or engage in masturbation during work hours. Some individuals may be terminated from their positions for engaging in these activities at work. They may miss time to either engage in the addiction or to deal with the legal repercussions of addiction-related activities.

CHANGES IN SOCIAL LIFE—Most sexual addicts can continue to have normal relationships with others, provided the addiction is not discovered. The addiction can affect the addict's social life as they pull away from friends and significant others. At times, sexual addicts may cross verbal and physical boundaries, making inappropriate comments or gestures that can interfere with social relationships. In cases where the addiction is discovered, social ties could be drastically affected or even terminated.

LYING—Sexual addicts, like any other addicts, will lie about the addiction, the time they spend involved in the addiction, and the reasons why they are avoiding family members or shirking responsibilities.

ACCOUNTABILITY ISSUES—In the earlier stages of the addiction, sexual addicts tend to be accountable regarding their responsibilities. As the addiction progresses, however, it is not uncommon for the time spent in the addiction to increase and their focus on executing responsibilities to decrease.

PERSONALITY CHANGES—Sex addicts become driven by their addiction. They can become more protective about their lives, neglect relationships with significant others, become emotionally distant, and experience mood swings. Their sexual behavior with their partner may also change, becoming either more intense or almost nonexistent.

ANGER AND VIOLENCE—Only in extreme cases of sexual addictions, such as sadomasochistic behaviors, do sexual addicts become angry or violent. They may exhibit some anger if their addiction is discovered, and they must attempt to defend or deny their actions.

COLLATERAL DAMAGE

The collateral damage often experienced as a result of a sexual addiction is twofold. First, by indulging in the addiction, the addicts themselves experience changes in their lives ranging from obsessive thoughts about sex, physical problems such as genital injury and sexually transmitted diseases, arrests, fines and other financial costs, shame, guilt, and secrecy.

Family members are the second recipients of the collateral damage. As the addict continues to indulge in the addiction, they may pull away from family members emotionally and physically. Family members may also be on the receiving end of any financial problems and may experience shame and humiliation should the addict's addiction become public knowledge. In extreme cases, family members may experience inappropriate comments, and in some cases, they may experience sexual abuse at the hands of the addict. In many cases, this behavior is perpetrated by individuals who, themselves, have been sexually traumatized.

SUMMING IT UP

Sex is a normal and necessary part of most people's lives. Engaging in sexual activity is a normal human function. The concern is when it moves into inappropriate areas and when it develops into an obsession that can have a serious impact on the life of the addict and those close to them.

All addictions feature obsessive-compulsive tendencies. Sexual addiction is no exception. Addiction changes lives, and sexual addiction, though it is one of the most closely guarded addictions, changes the lives of the addict and those close to them, including the sex addict, even before anyone realizes the addiction exists. Sexual addiction can be used as a coping device for some as they attempt to address challenging circumstances in their lives. In other cases, it may be learned behavior, particularly for those who were either sexually abused when they were young or who are raised in families where there was sexual dysfunction. In some cases, it is simply the activity that a person predisposed to addiction attaches themselves to.

So many sex addicts engage in voyeurism and pornography. In more serious cases, exhibitionism (exposing oneself to another person, often children) may be part of one's addiction. Pornography is viewed as harmless. However, it does run the risk of negatively impacting intimate relationships with significant others as the addict replaces those relationships with sexually addictive viewing practices. Exhibitionism may be connected to other mental health disorders. Be quick to report any incidences of exhibitionism to authorities.

Regardless of the cause of the addiction, like any other addiction, sexual addiction does affect the addict's life and the lives of those around them. Sex and sexual drives are a normal part of human development and behavior. Still, they can develop into obsessive-compulsive disorder that can jeopardize the healthy lives of the addicts and people close to them. Learning to understand the dynamics of one's sexual addiction and getting help from trained professionals can help a sexual addict recover from the dysfunctional aspects of their sex life. This can help them learn to live a life that is not dominated by sexual gratification and one that can be healthy and shared with those significant people in their lives.

If you or a family member are dealing with a sex addiction, call the Sex Addiction Hotline at (855) 945-4310.

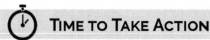

TIME TO TAKE ACTION

1. Solving any human problem starts with getting the necessary information to explain the problem's dynamics and progression. You can begin your fact-finding about sexual addiction with Internet searches, and there are many books available on the subject. If the facts you are gathering or the information you are reading in this chapter suggests that you or a family member may have a sexual addiction, don't wait. Get help quickly.

2. If you are experiencing obsessive and compulsive thoughts and behaviors about one of the forms of sexual addiction discussed earlier, start by talking to someone who has expertise in the area. There are counselors skilled in treating sexual addictions. If you are unsure where to find one, start with your primary- care physician.

3. If you are a family member of someone who has a sexual addiction, the advice is the same. Contact a counselor skilled in dealing with sexual addictions. You can also start with your family physician.

4. If you feel as though you may be dealing with a sexual addiction and it is affecting you and or your family, or you are the family member of someone who may be dealing with a sexual addiction, you can also call the number listed above.

DRIVING IT HOME

Human beings are physical organisms, and the drive for sex is programmed into our DNA. A healthy life also has a healthy sexual component or is the result of a conscious decision to abstain from sex, as may be the case for spiritual purposes or medical reasons). However, for some people, obsessions about sex and compulsive activity related to aspects of sexuality that are not productive can negatively impact their lives. They can damage relationships and affect one's feelings about oneself, causing guilt, shame, and, if the addiction is discovered, embarrassment. Family members may also find themselves dealing with shame and embarrassment if the addict's behavior becomes public knowledge. At the very least, it affects the loving and warm relationships that should exist in one's family. If you have a sexual addiction, or someone in your family does, be honest about it and get help.

YOUR DECLARATION IS: *I will learn to understand my sexual addiction, get help for it, and learn how to live a healthy sexual life!*

 ## ONWARD

In the next chapter, I will discuss how self-abuse begins as an instrument of control and diversion and develops into a cycle of self-abuse and addiction. I will discuss the addictive process that can develop through chronic periods of self-abusive behaviors.

CHAPTER 15

Self-Harm—From Control to Obsession

It begins as a way to cope with trauma and escape reality, but it can become an unrelenting and tormenting way of life.

PROCESSES TO EMPLOY: Brutal Honesty, I Over E, Present-Understand-Fix, Slowing Down Life's Pace, Internal Focus, Fact-Finding, Honesty, Slowing Down Life's Pace, Internal Focus, Patience, Truth-Telling, Belief, Listening, Trust

---

SELF-HARM REFERS TO WHEN A PERSON who has experienced past pain and trauma begins to hurt their own body on purpose. It is more common among women than men. For more details, see https://pubmed.ncbi.nlm.nih.gov/35698453/. A person who self-harms usually does not mean to kill themselves, but they are at higher risk of attempting suicide and dying by suicide if they do not receive help. Clinically known as nonsuicidal self-injury (NSSI), it is characterized by deliberate self-inflicted harm. People who self-harm may carve or cut their skin, burn themselves, beat or punch objects or themselves, embed objects under their skin, or engage in myriad other behaviors intended to cause themselves pain but not end their lives.

Examples of self-harm include:

➤ Cutting one's skin with a sharp object

➤ Piercing the skin with sharp objects

- Hitting or punching oneself or punching things (like a wall)
- Burning oneself with cigarettes, matches, or candles
- Deliberately breaking bones or bruising oneself
- Head banging on objects or hard surfaces
- Hair pulling

Self-harm tends to begin in teens or early adult years. Some people may engage in self-harm a few times and then stop. Others do it more often and have trouble stopping. For many people, self-harm gives them a sense of relief and is used to cope with a problem. Some teens say that when they hurt themselves, they are trying to stop feeling lonely, angry, or hopeless or to divert their attention from emotional pain.

Some reasons people may intentionally harm themselves are:

- To manage or reduce severe distress and provide a sense of relief.
- To help deal with severe trauma in one's life.
- To provide a distraction from painful emotions through physical pain.
- To deal with anxiety and depression.
- To feel a sense of control over one's body, feelings, or life situations.
- To address feelings of shame and guilt.
- To feel something, even if it is physical pain when feeling emotionally empty.
- To express internal feelings externally.
- To cope with feelings of loneliness and abandonment.
- To communicate feelings of stress or depression to the outside world.
- To punish oneself.
- Because it has become an addiction.

THE STATISTICS

It is difficult to compile statistics related to self-harm because very few people report the behavior, and even through self-reports, the acts are minimized in severity and quantity. A small representation of some of these statistics that have been reported are:[16]

1. 7.7% of early adolescents reported engaging in NSSI.

2. 13.9% to 21.4% of high school adolescents (grades 9–12, average age 16) reported engaging in NSSI.

3. In college-age samples, rates of NSSI can be as high as 38%.

Many people who self-harm either stumble upon self-harm accidentally, such as experiencing a cut on their finger or arm, being burned with something hot, or a shallow piercing from a sharp object. When this happens, they may have experienced relief or distraction from a stressful or traumatic event, stress or depression, bullying, and abuse, or personal or family conditions that cause them to experience shame, guilt, or low self-esteem.

Most who self-harm feel as though all or most of their life is out of their control. Self-harm can give them control over one aspect of their lives, and since typically no one knows what they are doing, they can perform the act anytime they want to, and doing so provides relief from the pain they feel is defining their lives.

Cutting oneself with a blade or other sharp object is the most prevalent form of self-harm. Cuts are typically made on the arms, wrists, ankles, and thighs. Other body parts may be used, with the defining approach being to cut in areas that are not visible to other people. Sometimes, the cuts are deep, though most of the time, they are superficial. The goal is to experience a degree of initial pain that their brains interpret as soothing while diverting their attention from other painful parts of their lives. People will also pierce their skin with sharp objects, usually in the same places as those who use cutting.

Typically, the more drastic forms of self-harm are used to cope with more severe pain and trauma. For example, the individual may cut deeper when shallow cutting isn't working. Also, forms of self-harm like burning oneself with cigarettes or breaking bones are usually used to cope with more traumatic and painful life circumstances or when the milder forms of self-harm are not relieving their symptoms. These more drastic ways of inflicting harm on oneself could also be associated with more severe mental health concerns such as schizophrenia. Still, if one uses them, it does not necessarily mean they have deep psychological problems.

Adolescent females are more likely to use self-harm methods than their male counterparts. See https://www.sciencedirect.com/science/article/pii/S0165032723012995. The behavior can sometimes subside, especially when life circumstances are less severe. However, for some people, the behavior will continue through adolescence and into the early twenties. Still, for others, the behavior could progress and remain active well into the thirties, and, in some cases, beyond.

Of particular concern is the addictive potential for self-harm. As the brain begins to accommodate the behavior, as with all other addictions, it will push the addict to perform the self-harming act simply because an addiction has developed. Self-harm addiction may continue regardless of the extent of physical injuries, hospitalizations, and collateral damage.

Symptoms and warning signs of self-harm include:

➤ Scars, usually on body parts that can be hidden under clothing

➤ Wearing long sleeves or pants, even in hot weather

➤ Talking about feeling worthless or helpless

➤ Fresh cuts, bruises, bite marks, burns, or injured bones

➤ Keeping sharp objects on hand

➤ Frequent reports of accidental injury

➤ Emotional and behavioral instability and unpredictability

➤ Increased isolation from family members and friends

➤ Mood swings and depression

➤ Patches of hair loss

➤ Unexplained scars or other injuries

THE PROGRESSION

1. The person is having a difficult time managing stress, may be feeling out of control, or might be dealing with depression, past issues of abuse, or other circumstances that cause them to feel emotional pain

2. Nothing they have tried is relieving their emotional pain.

3. The person hears how someone else is relieving their emotional pain by hurting themselves, or they have an experience such as cutting, poking oneself, or burning, and feel some relief or pleasure from the experience.

4. In this first experience with inadvertent self-harm, the person feels relief from one or more of the stressors in their life.

5. The person performs the behavior for a second time and, once again, feels the same relief they felt after the first episode.

6. The person performs the behavior a third time and decides that continued indulgence in the behavior could help reduce stress and other problems in their life.

7. The person begins to experiment with other forms of self-harm to determine which might be the best to help them feel better.

8. The person decides on a particular method, which might be cutting, poking, burning, pulling hair, or breaking bones, and continues to secretly perform the behavior now as a ritual to help feel in control and to divert attention away from emotional pain.

9. When questioned about marks, cuts, or any other indicators of bodily harm, the person lies and tells others that they accidentally hurt themselves.

10. The person begins to cover up body parts where the self-harm is being administered.

11. As the person continues the behavior, their brains adjust to the pain.

12. As the behavior becomes emotionally accepted and the body adjusts to increasing pain levels, it becomes a routine part of life.

13. Now, developing a tolerance for the behavior, the individual begins to self-harm even when there are no intellectual or emotional stressors to offset.

14. Now addicted to the behavior, the self-harm addict continues to perform the behaviors without any concern for consequences.

15. Lying and protective behaviors increase, and the addict becomes more defensive against others' attempts to stop the behavior.

16. The addict fantasizes about self-harm behaviors and has a daily plan to continue performing them.

17. When the addict does not have the opportunity to perform the behaviors, they will experience withdrawal behaviors such as intolerance, anger, and panic.

18. In extreme cases of withdrawal, the addict can experience physical symptoms that mirror those experienced by drug addicts, such as nausea, headaches, and body aches.

19. In cases when the addict does physical damage during self-harm behaviors, doctor visits and hospitalizations can occur.

20. Regardless of the damage to the body, opinions of others, enhanced secrecy, social rejection, or family issues, the addict remains steadfast regarding their continued self-harm behaviors.

21. In more intense cases, self-harm behaviors can result in permanent physical damage, and in some extreme cases, the addict may lose their life.

IN THE CLUTCHES

No addiction is free from the problems and side effects that develop from continued use. What follows is a list of the effects that one can experience from addiction to any drug or activity. Different addictions can lead to different problems, as you will see as we continue.

PHYSICAL PROBLEMS—The addict suffers damage to the skin, veins, and bones, infections, damage to hair follicles, and permanent scarring.

MENTAL HEALTH ISSUES—The self-harm addict grapples with sensations of guilt, shame, secrecy, isolation, and feeling dirty, as well as depression, anxiety, and self-esteem issues.

COMMUNICATION PROBLEMS—Communication is affected as secrecy and isolation develop. Self-harm addicts can become defensive and evasive and blame others for their problems.

LEGAL PROBLEMS—Typically, there are no legal problems associated with self-harm.

FINANCIAL CONCERNS—Financial problems associated with self-harm are usually related to medical expenses associated with doctor visits and hospitalizations.

FAMILY AND RELATIONSHIP ISSUES—As communication decreases and secrecy develops, the addict can pull away from other family members. However, since self-harm can help a person feel better for a short time, there are periods when they are connected to other family members. As the addiction becomes more prominent, however, family relationships can suffer as family members do their best to stop the addict from hurting themselves, and the addict continues to defend the addiction.

EMPLOYMENT PROBLEMS—The problems associated with employment occur when the addict is either injured or hospitalized as a result of severe self-harm or when they self-harm at work.

CHANGES IN SOCIAL LIFE—As long as the addict can hide any visible signs of self-harm, social life does not change appreciably. However, as the addiction continues to become more established in the addict's life, they may pull away from friends and spend more time alone in emotionally safe locations.

LYING—Consistent with other addictions, self-harm addicts will lie to protect not only their addiction but other aspects of their life, especially when confrontations might lead to a loss of control, reliving old traumas, and emotional and/or physical vulnerability on the part of the addict.

ACCOUNTABILITY ISSUES—Accountability is not as much associated with the self-harm behavior as it is with the symptoms that cause it. Issues like depression, anxiety, self-esteem, mood swings, anger, resentment, and rumination may occur because of past pain and trauma, and it is these issues that affect accountability.

PERSONALITY CHANGES—Since, in many cases, self-harm can stem from childhood trauma, abuse, and unresolved issues, mood swings can develop, and with the addiction only addressing the symptoms of the problem and not the cause, conditions like anxiety, depression, and low self-esteem can persist. In more severe cases, borderline personality issues may develop or be exacerbated.

ANGER AND VIOLENCE—Often, in the initial stages, self-harm may reduce anger; however, as the addiction progresses and withdrawal becomes part of the dynamics of the addiction, mood swings will continue, and anger can be displayed. In more severe cases, violence can result and be directed at others as they challenge the addict's behavior or as the self-harm behaviors fail to make the addict feel better.

COLLATERAL DAMAGE

While the self-harm addict may be successful in diverting their attention away from past pain and trauma, the cost to themselves can be significant. The secrecy that surrounds the behavior must be maintained to avoid confrontation with family members and significant others who may try to stop them from continuing to hurt themselves. In addition, the harm they are doing to their bodies can be severe and have long-lasting negative effects.

Family members may find themselves exposed to the personality changes that accompany self-harm, such as isolation, protectiveness, anxiety, and depression, and the secrecy designed to help support the addiction. When family members do identify that the addict is hurting themselves, they will do everything in their power to stop it, and this often puts significant emotional strain on already difficult relationships.

Family members may attempt to bring in outside help, such as doctors and counselors, and this usually increases the anger the addict will experience as they perceive that their control over what they are doing is being robbed from them. As the addiction progresses, family members may need to become involved in individual and family counseling programs with the addict. The addict may require visits to medical doctors and, in more drastic cases, hospitalizations either for the physical damage they are inflicting on themselves or for mental health reasons. The stress and worry that family members experience can progress to the point that they, themselves, need counseling services.

SUMMING IT UP

It is crucial to understand the addictive potential of self-harm behaviors. I have discussed habit formation in this book and every book in The Fix Yourself Empowerment Series. Our bodies and minds adjust to what they are presented with, whether they instigate positive or negative circumstances. As people who inflict self-harm on themselves continue with these behaviors, the body and the mind do adjust, and addiction is a strong possibility.

Get to know the symptoms and warning signs of self-harm. They are listed earlier in this chapter. Intervention has less to do with stopping the self-harm behaviors and more to do with understanding the underlying causes of the problems. Please pay attention to the progression of the addiction and try not to be critical or angry with a family member who may be hurting themselves. Don't try to stop this on your own. Let professionals with training in self-harm help you. This is a condition that, though difficult to treat, is not impossible with the right intervention.

You can start things by calling (866) 488-7386 or texting the crisis hotline at 741741.

TIME TO TAKE ACTION

1. Take some time to understand the dynamics of self-harm. This will help you take the correct steps to help someone who may be hurting themselves.

2. If you are performing self-harm rituals, know that you are only treating the symptoms. Be willing to get help. Call 1-866-488-7386 or text 741741.

3. Counseling programs are often quite successful in treating people who are suffering from the pain and past traumas that lead to self-harm behaviors. By contacting the confidential number above, you can be referred to someone who can help you without anyone else finding out about your addiction.

4. If you are a family member or a significant person in the life of someone who is harming themselves, try to refrain from attacking only the behaviors. The addict may perceive your intentions as harmful. Try to understand that they have a problem, be willing to support them, validate that they do have pain in their lives, and try to help them move in the direction of intervention. Start with a visit to your primary care physician to address any physical issues that may have developed from the self-harm and for a referral for additional help.

 ## DRIVING IT HOME

Much of the attention given to self-harm is directed toward the damage the person is doing to themselves. Therapeutic measures are often designed to treat past traumas, control issues, and other emotional concerns. It is not often that we see treatment approaches directed toward self-harm as an addiction. However, as one's mind and the body adjust to this coping mechanism as a way to relieve pain and divert attention away from emotionally difficult situations, these behaviors can easily develop into addictions that can direct the course of one's life. If you are harming yourself to address past pains and traumas, it is so important that you get help before this coping device takes control of your life.

YOUR DECLARATION IS: *I will be honest about my self-harm, and I will get help to address the root causes of this behavior!*

 ONWARD

In the next chapter, I will discuss shopaholics, why they do what they do, and the neurotic/depressive/obsessive need to continue chasing the quick fixes that never fix anything but, in the end, can destroy everything.

◇◇◇◇◇◇◇◇◇◇◇◇◇◇

CHAPTER 16

Shopping—Quick Fix, Small Reward

It is the tantalizing trap adorned with glitter and excitement.
It can become the bottomless pit on a never-ending acquisition
merry-go-round.

PROCESSES TO EMPLOY: Brutal Honesty, I Over E, Present-Understand-Fix, Slowing Down Life's Pace, Internal Focus, Fact-Finding, Honesty, Slowing Down Life's Pace, Internal Focus, Patience, Truth-Telling, Belief, Listening, Trust

---

SHOPAHOLICS HAVE A COMPULSION TO SHOP. Such people engage in compulsive buying as a way to feel good either about themselves or the conditions of their lives and avoid negative feelings such as anxiety and depression. Some people use compulsive shopping as a substitute for attention, affection, nurturance, and love. It is arguably the most socially acceptable type of addiction.

The clinical name for compulsive shopping is "oniomania," defined as *an abnormal impulse to buy things or a condition characterized by such impulses.* It is easy to defend compulsive shopping since, in developed cultures, shopping is how we stock our shelves and obtain all the resources we need to stay alive and add comfort to our lives. In this manner, it is similar to food addictions since we need food to survive. Likewise, unless one lives completely off the grid, shopping is the process we use to obtain what we need.

THE STATISTICS

There are high rates of comorbidities (the simultaneous presence of two or more diseases or medical conditions in a patient) with shopping addiction. Research from the University of Iowa reported that 84% of young adults who suffer from shopping addiction report a family history of mental health disorders, such as mood or anxiety disorders. Respondents in the study with shopping addiction were found to have the following comorbidities:[17]

1. Mood disorders (21%–100%)

2. Anxiety disorders (41%–80%)

3. Substance use disorders (21–46%)

4. Eating disorders (8–35%)

The signs that a person might have a shopping addiction include:

➤ Always thinking about items they plan to purchase

➤ Being unable to stop their compulsive shopping

➤ Experiencing a rush during and after buying something

➤ Feeling regret or guilt about things they have purchased

➤ Financial problems or an inability to pay off debts

➤ Lying about things they have bought or hiding their purchases

➤ Opening new credit cards without paying off balances on existing cards

➤ Regularly purchasing things they don't need or already have

Compulsive shopping is a quick-fix behavior. It is something a person knows can temporarily fix the way they feel. While they are shopping, there is an exhilaration not unlike what a gambler feels while gambling. One of the myths about shopaholics is that they shop to accumulate more resources, such as clothing, electronics, and household goods. However, it is not what is purchased that changes their mood or temporarily changes the conditions of their lives. The acquisition process—that is, the buying experience—does the trick and also creates the addiction.

The addictive process of shopping has the same effect on the brain as any other addiction. It raises neurotransmitter levels and creates euphoria, providing that quick-fix change that can improve mood and negative feelings. It is the change in neurology that begins the addictive process, and as it continues to develop, what began as an enjoyable afternoon activity progresses to a compulsion and finally to an addiction.

THE PROGRESSION

1. The person shops sporadically, usually to purchase items they or their family may need.

2. While shopping, the person buys small pleasure items to add to the shopping list.

3. Enjoying pleasure, the person continues buying similar items.

4. The person looks for sales and adds to the "comfort items."

5. The person begins to notice that when they shop, they are not thinking about problems in their lives, are less depressed or anxious, and are having a good time.

6. The person begins to shop more often, usually in shopping centers, clothing stores, and shopping malls.

7. Shopping expands to online purchases, though this type of shopping does not produce the same euphoria as malls and shopping centers.

8. The person begins to exceed their budget and is charging more on their credit cards.

9. As the credit card bills arrive, other family members, usually their significant other, confront them about the increased bills.

10. The person lies and says it was for needed items, maybe for the children, or that some purchases are being returned and the charge will be removed from the credit card.

11. As shopping moves into the addictive phase, the addict shops more often and buys more items. Many of them will never be used.

12. The addict, experiencing more anger from loved ones or significant others, continues to shop and lies to cover the problem.

13. Credit card companies and bill collectors begin calling, and the addict ignores the calls.

14. As is common, debt collectors begin to call the addict's family members. Meanwhile, the addict's credit cards are being maxed out.

15. The addict opens new credit cards without settling the old ones and begins charging on those.

16. Significant others are complaining about the bills, the impact on credit ratings, and the addict's unwillingness to stop charging.

17. Family members take steps to remove themselves from debt, and the addict is running out of resources to continue the process.

18. As with many addictions, shopping addicts will lie and, if necessary, steal to obtain the funds to continue with the addiction.

19. Even with the threat of divorce or legal action, the shopaholic continues to shop.

20. Now faced with severe family and financial problems, the addict's shopping is drastically reduced.

21. The addict goes into withdrawal, and the initial symptoms, such as depression, anxiety, and past and current personal problems, intensify.

22. The addict looks for ways to make peace with other people but continues with the addiction.

Though there is more social acceptance for shopping addiction than other addictions, it can have a tremendous impact on family finances and relationships. It is not uncommon for family members to pay off the shopaholic's debts with the promise from the addict that they will discontinue the shopping. However, many of them return to the addictive shopping, and once again, the credit card bills begin to mount.

As is the case in any addiction, it is unwise to accept the addict's promises. Paying off credit cards and smoothing over difficult family situations does nothing more than treat addictive symptoms and enable the addict. It is important to get to the causes of the problem. In some cases, it will simply be an addictive personality that has attached itself to shopping. In other cases, it is depression, anxiety, and other personal problems that drive the addiction. If these traumatic intellectual and emotional undercurrents are not treated, it will be difficult for a shopping addict to change their behavior.

IN THE CLUTCHES

No addiction is free from the problems and side effects that develop from continued use. What follows is a list of the effects that one can experience from addiction to any drug or activity. Different addictions can lead to different problems, as you will see as we continue.

PHYSICAL PROBLEMS—There are no physical problems that are directly associated with shopping addiction.

MENTAL HEALTH ISSUES—Mental health issues remain the same as before the addiction began. They are typically anxiety, depression, unhappiness with current life situations, and past traumas and pain.

COMMUNICATION PROBLEMS—Communication problems develop as the addict continues to spend and finances become a problem. These typically take the form of arguments and communication shutdowns.

LEGAL PROBLEMS—Legal problems can develop as debt climbs. At times, court actions may be involved, retailers may file charges for bad checks, and charges may be filed against the addict. for using credit cards that may not belong to the addict. Charges can also be filed for theft, receiving, shoplifting, and fraud.

FINANCIAL CONCERNS—In the early stages of shopping, finances may be impacted but not significantly. As the addiction progresses, debt is incurred, credit cards are maxed out, bank accounts may be drained, and, in serious cases, bankruptcies may be filed.

FAMILY AND RELATIONSHIP ISSUES—As shopping bills become excessive, family relationships become strained, and in some cases, the addiction may lead to separation and divorce.

EMPLOYMENT PROBLEMS—There are no employment problems that are specifically associated with shopping addiction. Shopping addicts may even work longer hours to obtain the funds they need to support their addiction. Also, they may make short trips to the store, only to return to work late.

CHANGES IN SOCIAL LIFE—There are usually no changes in shopping addicts' social life. They may even shop with friends and build all or part of their social life around their shopping addiction.

LYING—Lying is an integral part of shopping addiction. Addicts lie about what they purchase, how much time they spend shopping, and how much money they spend. In addition, they may lie about how they are securing the funds to continue with the addiction.

ACCOUNTABILITY ISSUES—Shoppers remain accountable in the addiction's early stages. However, as shopping time and financial expenditures increase, responsibilities can be avoided or left undone.

PERSONALITY CHANGES—As the addiction proceeds to the more advanced stages, anxiety and depression will return, along with family problems and financial debt. The addict will also experience periods of shame, guilt, and victimization.

ANGER AND VIOLENCE—There is typically no violence associated with shopping addiction; however, as the addiction progresses, anger may become part of the process as significant others confront the addict, and the addict does whatever is possible to defend the addiction.

COLLATERAL DAMAGE

Compulsive shopping is nothing but a quick fix, and quick fixes rarely, if ever, work. For a short time, depression, anxiety, and other stressors are put aside, and the addict enjoys the rush that comes with the shopping experience. However, when the shopping spree ends, the addict will return to the same symptoms that drove them to the compulsive behavior. They will again become anxious, depressed, or dissatisfied, and they may add new problems to their already unhappy way of life. As this unrealistic behavior continues, they will experience guilt, shame, and embarrassment.

Family members are forced to be part of a downward financial ride that often includes draining savings accounts and taking out loans to settle overwhelming debts the shopping addict has accumulated. Relationships can be destroyed as family members watch so much of what they worked so hard to accomplish being irresponsibly spent at the hands of the addicted family member. In addition to the debt that must be paid and depleted savings, liens may be taken out on homes; debt collectors come calling, credit ratings plummet, and, in some cases, bankruptcy and criminal charges result from this irresponsible way of life.

SUMMING IT UP

Shopping may be considered a more accepted form of compulsive behavior, but it is not innocent. The damage to finances, families, businesses, and mental health can be staggering. Since compulsive shopping can fall under the guise of an accepted behavior, it is often, except in extraordinary cases, not thought of as a true addiction. However, it possesses so many of the characteristics of serious addictions.

Shopping addiction, like any other addiction, does not allow the time for rational thought and concerns about consequences and collateral damage. Addicts obsess about shopping and will continue to engage in the behavior long after their finances have been damaged or drained.

There is no such thing as an acceptable addiction. Every addiction has consequences, and every addiction takes prisoners. Shopping addiction is no exception. Recovery from shopping addiction is possible, but trying to do it on your own is rarely successful. The advice is to treat this like any addiction, be honest about it, and get help for it.

You can find help for a shopping addiction at Shoppers Anonymous. Find them at https://debtorsanonymous.org/. Everything is confidential.

 TIME TO TAKE ACTION

1. Never underestimate the power of a shopping addiction. If you have the signs and symptoms presented earlier in the chapter, it is important to get help before this addiction destroys your finances, your life, and the lives of those you love. Call the helpline above.

2. Shopping addiction is easy to rationalize. It is important to be honest about this. If you have the signs and symptoms, be willing to admit it. Recovery from this devastating addiction starts by admitting there's a problem.

3. If a family member has a shopping addiction, do not enable what they are doing. This needs to be addressed head-on. Your first concern is to protect your finances. Ensure the addict does not have access to the funds you need to run your home, savings accounts, checkbook, and credit cards.

4. If your family member has a shopping addiction and is unwilling to stop, talk to an attorney to determine what you need to do to protect yourself financially and legally.

Driving It Home

No addiction should be taken for granted. Any of them can turn you into a slave to compulsive behavior, tear families apart, and, in this and many other cases, wreck your finances. Sensible shopping must be done to stock the shelves and procure the resources needed to survive and be happy. Shopping addiction pushes far past the boundaries of sensible shopping. It has all the characteristics of other addictions. It is so important not to treat this one lightly or enable it in any fashion. Treat it for what it is: an addiction. Support groups and counseling are available. Don't wait until your shopping addiction has destroyed your finances. Get help now.

YOUR DECLARATION IS: *I will treat my compulsive shopping as an addiction, and I will get the help I need to restore my life to sanity!*

 ## Onward

In the next chapter, I will discuss workaholism, which is the need to continue overinvesting oneself in work and work-related functions. I will examine where this behavior begins, how it develops, and what keeps people slaves to their work lives.

◇◇◇◇◇◇◇◇◇◇◇◇◇

CHAPTER 17

Workaholism— Constructive Destruction

From working to live to living to work. It's a never-ending destructive cycle that disconnects you from your world.

PROCESSES TO EMPLOY: Brutal Honesty, I Over E, Present-Understand-Fix, Slowing Down Life's Pace, Honesty, Focus, Patience, Truth-Telling, Belief, Listening, Trust

---

WORKAHOLISM IS CHARACTERIZED BY WORKING EXCESSIVE HOURS (beyond workplace or financial requirements), thinking continually about work, and a lack of work enjoyment unrelated to actual workplace demands. For some, it is an all-consuming obsessive-compulsive disorder.

Workaholism may be seen as a prerequisite for success. Consequently, some individuals may find it extremely difficult to stop working, even when they are allowed to do so. Workaholism is associated with reduced physical health and various psychiatric disorders, including anxiety, attention-deficit/hyperactivity disorder (ADHD), depression, and obsessive-compulsive disorder (OCD).

Signs and symptoms of workaholism are:

➤ Having a hard time stopping work

➤ Working unnecessarily long hours

➤ Talking about nothing but work

- Working to reduce guilt and anxiety

- Constantly thinking about work

- Intense fear of failure

- A neglected personal life

- Work-related perfectionism

- Sacrificing personal time for work

- Less time spent in intimate relationships

- Difficulty enjoying time away from work

- Routinely working longer than one's colleagues

- Taking on unnecessary part-time jobs

Workaholism may begin as a way to escape from personal problems like relationship issues, health problems, tight finances, and past traumas and pain. Similar to shopping addiction, society doesn't stigmatize workaholism. Working long hours is considered one of the characteristics of an exemplary employee. Employees are often rewarded for going above and beyond in the workplace, for the appearance of loyalty to the company, and for being willing to work longer hours, often taking on double shifts, and rarely taking time off.

THE STATISTICS

Here are recent statistics on workaholism:[18]

1. Workaholics work an average of 62 hours per week.

2. Approximately 10% of the U.S. population identify as workaholics.

3. Workaholics have a 33% higher risk of stroke.

4. 69% of workaholics exhibit signs of physical and mental health decline.

5. Workaholics are three times more likely to suffer from depression.

6. Workaholics are 19% more likely to miss their children's important events.

7. 48% of workaholics have clinical insomnia.

8. Workaholics are 50% more likely to skip vacations.

9. They may forfeit paid time off

10. Workaholics are 34% more likely to report poor health than non-workaholics.

11. Workaholics are 45% more likely to suffer from heart attacks.

12. 32% of workaholics suffer from intense headaches due to stress.

13. Workaholics have a 70% higher risk of diabetes.

14. 81% of workaholics said they struggle with work-life balance.

15. Workaholics are twice as likely to suffer from anxiety.

As is the case in other addictions, workaholism begins as a healthy commitment to doing a good job and bringing home a good paycheck. What makes workaholism different from other addictions, however, is that employers, supervisors, other employees, and society in general can see it as a positive attribute and reward the behavior. Accolades like employee of the month, earning considerable bonuses, and promotions all come with dedication to the job, and workaholics excel in job excellence, attendance, and extended time on the job. What makes workaholism similar to other addictions is that it consumes an individual's time and energy to the point that it affects so many other areas of their lives. As it progresses into an addiction, there is a profound effect on relationships and homebound responsibilities.

THE PROGRESSION

1. The person acquires a job and does their best to be considered a quality employee.

2. The employee learns every aspect of the job and strives to impress supervisors with their efficiency and dedication.

3. When asked to work overtime, the employee gladly accepts the offer.

4. The employee learns the responsibilities of additional positions with the company and fills in when other employees are away.

5. The employee begins to ask for overtime, even though it may not be financially necessary.

6. When the employee is not at work, they consistently think about work-related activities and how to work more efficiently when they return.

7. Some responsibilities are either not done at home or neglected as additional time is spent on work-related activities.

8. The employee brings suggestions into work to help things run more efficiently there.

9. The employee is rewarded with a promotion for outstanding commitment to the company.

10. With the increased responsibilities, the employee spends more time at work, often working longer hours, filling in on weekends, and sometimes working double shifts.

11. Family and significant others complain about the time the person spends at work.

12. The employee continues to increase their evolvement at work and is having difficulty taking days off.

13. Relationship issues begin, and spouses and significant others make their concerns known to the workaholic.

14. The workaholic employee becomes defensive, rationalizing their work obsession by saying it provides the family with a higher standard of living.

15. The workaholic does less around the house, does not attend family activities, and neglects intimate relationships in favor of increased work time and obsessive thinking about work during off hours.

16. Family members begin talking about the person's job in terms of an addiction or the person's "lover."

17. Now addicted to the work environment, the addict vehemently defends their actions and becomes angry when challenged about work-related concerns.

18. Their loved ones and significant others are beginning to give ultimatums if the behavior does not change.

19. The addict assures Their loved ones and significant others that they will make some changes, but this either does not happen or the changes are short-lived.

20. When the addict is not involved in work or work-related activities, they can become restless and temperamental.

21. Home-related responsibilities can help the addict fill some of the off-work hours, but these activities do not provide the emotional rush the addict receives at work.

22. Despite the objections of family and significant others, the work addict continues to work long hours and remains consumed with work-related activities.

23. Significant others may respond by extramarital affairs, separations, and even filing for divorce.

24. The addict is unable to alter the work-related behavior and promises to change but can never follow through and make the necessary changes.

25. The addict is defensive, blames others for the problems they are having, feels that they are ungrateful for how much the addict is doing for them, is miserable when they are not working, and continues to find ways to remain overly involved with work and work-related responsibilities.

Since workaholism is often met with much positive reinforcement from employers, there is a fine line between the negative consequences of an addiction and the positive reinforcement that comes with being an excellent employee. This makes workaholism a difficult addiction to diagnose and also to change. Even scheduling a day off becomes difficult for the work addict. They firmly believe that reducing their involvement in their job will negatively impact their lives. Also, when they are not at work, they experience the same withdrawal other addicts experience when their "drug of choice" is absent from their lives.

IN THE CLUTCHES

No addiction is free from the problems and side effects that develop from continued use. What follows is a list of the effects that one can experience from addiction to any drug or activity. Different addictions can lead to different problems, as you will see as we continue.

PHYSICAL PROBLEMS—Workaholism taxes the body by way of sleep problems, physical exhaustion, head and body aches, fatigue, exacerbated ADD and ADHD, focusing and memory issues, and substance abuse.

MENTAL HEALTH ISSUES—Anxiety, depression, increased stress, emotional exhaustion, worry, perfectionism, obsessive-compulsive tendencies, and guilt frequently manifest with workaholism.

COMMUNICATION PROBLEMS—Work-related communication increases, but communication in the addict's personal life sufferers because the addict is often unavailable, usually exhausted, and focused on work-related concerns. Arguments with spouses and significant others increase, and the addict begins to avoid communicative confrontations. As intimacy issues increase, communication becomes strained and often expressed with anger.

LEGAL PROBLEMS—There are typically no legal issues associated with workaholism.

FINANCIAL CONCERNS—Workaholism causes no financial problems. Working extended hours usually increases one's income.

FAMILY AND RELATIONSHIP ISSUES—Relationships often suffer at the hands of the obsessive-compulsive nature of workaholism. There is a sharp reduction in time spent in relationships and at family functions, and family members feel as though work is more important to the addict than they are. There are typically issues with intimacy and affection, and family members can feel abandoned and rejected.

EMPLOYMENT PROBLEMS—There are rarely any problems with employment unless the addict becomes so hyper-focused at work that it interferes with their relationships with other employees.

CHANGES IN SOCIAL LIFE—There can be drastic changes in social life as the addict continues to spend more time at work. The workaholic will miss family functions and outside social activities. They are often unavailable to nurture social relationships.

LYING—Work addicts may lie to family and friends about having to go to work. They may lie about responsibilities not being performed at home and their willingness to reduce their time and commitment to their job.

ACCOUNTABILITY ISSUES—Workaholics are accountable for work, but beyond that, they have a difficult time with other responsibilities. They often cannot be counted on to attend family activities, get things done around the house, and be available for emotional support for family and significant others.

PERSONALITY CHANGES—Workaholics experience increases in obsessive-compulsive behaviors. They need to be perfect, can develop control issues, and often need approval from work-related supervisors. They are obsessive and may become more neurotic, especially about work-related concerns.

ANGER AND VIOLENCE—Since workaholism has an effect on sleep schedules and leads to exhaustion and fatigue, a workaholic can react quicker and more intensely in challenging situations. They can be verbally abusive and do not like to be challenged. In extreme cases, they can become violent, directing their violence primarily to objects, but at times, they may be violent with other people, especially if substance abuse is also involved.

COLLATERAL DAMAGE

Though commitment to work is often seen as a positive personal attribute, it can have a tremendous impact on the addict's personal life, family members, and other people in their lives. The work addict can experience significant increases in obsessive-compulsive behaviors, anger, exhaustion, and other stress-related concerns. They overprioritize their employment and often reduce their involvement in family-related relationships, social events with friends, and home-related responsibilities. They may overindulge in caffeine or other stimulants to help them keep up with responsibilities at work and the long hours that make up their day, and use other drugs like alcohol or marijuana to decompress.

Family members can feel abandoned and rejected and will voice their concerns about not being important in the work addict's life. Though finances are typically not an issue, intimate personal relationships suffer at the hands of the workaholic. The emotional welfare of the family does not seem to be a priority for the work addict, and family members are quick to let them know that.

Unable to see the big picture at home, workaholics feel taken for granted and firmly believe their actions are in the family's best interest. They do not recognize their compulsive work routine as an addiction and question how their family could have concerns about their willingness to give them a better life. Family members will respond by saying they need to spend more quality time with the addict. When this does not happen, it can lead to severe family stress and, in more severe cases, to the breakup of the family unit.

SUMMING IT UP

Workaholism is socially accepted in many cultures, enhances the financial stability of the family, and can increase the work addict's self-esteem. Unfortunately, as it progresses, workaholism can have a serious impact on the quality of life for the addict and their families. Regardless of how good it makes the person feel and of the increased financial stability it produces, workaholism is still an addiction, and every addiction has the power to destroy an addict's life and that of their loved ones.

Like any other addiction, workaholism causes increases in neuro-transmitter activity. It produces a euphoria that must be repeated consistently to maintain the euphoric state and to avoid the withdrawal that happens when the activity is absent from the addict's life. It's nice to be known as a hard worker who is engaged in the lives, responsibilities, and activities of one's family and who is also willing to sacrifice for the good of the company. It is something entirely different to lose oneself and one's family to an addiction that can consume everyone and everything in its path.

All too often, the workaholic must be taken to the brink of disaster before they make changes in their work life. By that time, considerable damage can be done, and in some cases, the damage may be irreversible. There is help for workaholism, and if treated early enough, the balance between work and family life can be restored, along with the relationships that are so important to everyone involved. If you think the balance between your work and family life is problematic, it makes sense to get help for your addiction.

You can start by calling Workaholics Anonymous (WA) at (512) 415-8468. The call is confidential and can provide resources to help you.

 TIME TO TAKE ACTION

1. You can also visit the WA website at Workaholics-Anonymous. org.

2. If someone in your family is a workaholic, it also makes good sense to contact a counselor to help you deal with this addiction. If you are unsure where to start, call Workaholics Anonymous (WA).

3. Make a list of all the things you need to do at home and in your personal life. If you are leaving them undone because you are over-committing to your work schedule, discuss the matter with family members. Be willing to listen to what they have to say.

4. Schedule a meeting with your employer to discuss your work schedule and the balance you need between it and your personal life.

5. Sometimes, workaholism is a symptom of other family or personal concerns. Family counseling is always a good idea to address work addiction and the issues it may be covering. A family counselor can help you with this.

 ## DRIVING IT HOME

It's important to understand workaholism for the addiction that it is. Every addiction can cause severe damage both to the addict and to family members. However, every addiction can be treated successfully, and lives can be restored to health and happiness. It is so important to establish a balance between your work life and your family life. Discussions about how much money is necessary to run the family home and serve family needs and how much time must be spent in the family and home settings are important parts of a healthy relationship. Take the time to discuss the priorities in your life and the balance needed to address those priorities. Take care of your work business, but also take the time to care for your family.

YOUR DECLARATION IS: *I will understand my workaholism as an addiction, and I will do what it takes to restore balance in my life!*

 ## ONWARD

In the next chapter, I will examine how exercise, like other drugs, causes a significant change in neurotransmitter production and how this can develop into an addictive process. I will also discuss how the exercise addict never seems to measure up to their ideal version of themselves and how this fuels this insidious, addictive way of living.

CHAPTER 18

Exercise Addiction— Never Measuring Up

It slowly attaches itself to your body, your emotions, and your mind. It tells you that you are never good enough.

PROCESSES TO EMPLOY: Brutal Honesty, I Over E, Present-Understand-Fix, Slowing Down Life's Pace, Internal Focus, Fact-Finding, Honesty, Slowing Down Life's Pace, Internal Focus, Patience, Truth-Telling, Belief, Listening, Trust

---

EXERCISE ADDICTION IS A COMPULSIVE DRIVE to engage in physical exercise despite negative consequences. Similar to other addictions, a person with exercise addiction may be aware of the negative impacts of their behavior but still proceed with excessive exercise with little concern for any consequences. Exercise can develop into an addiction for anyone, regardless of age, gender, race, intelligence, vocation, or physical condition.

The adage that says a body in motion stays in motion could not be more accurate. Physical exercise is necessary to become and stay healthy and to help maintain the balance that leads to a happy and productive life. Done in moderation and with realistic goals and an efficient workout program, exercise builds strength, sharpens the senses, serves as an emotional outlet, and increases the production of dopamine and endorphins. However, when it becomes a compulsion, it can become an antagonist to good health physically, emotionally, and intellectually.

In the article "How Much Is Too Much? The Development and Validation of the Exercise Addiction Scale," researchers Hausenblas and Downs identify exercise addiction based on the following seven criteria.[19] (these are modifications of the DSM-IV-TR criteria for substance dependence):

1. **TOLERANCE**: Increasing the amount of exercise to feel the desired effect, be it a" buzz" or a sense of accomplishment.

2. **WITHDRAWAL**: In the absence of exercise, the person experiences negative effects, such as anxiety, irritability, restlessness, and sleep problems.

3. **LACK OF CONTROL**: Unsuccessful attempts to reduce exercise level or cease exercising for a specified amount of time.

4. **INTENTION EFFECTS**: Inability to stick to one's intended routine, as evidenced by exceeding the amount of time devoted to exercise or consistently exceeding the intended amount.

5. **TIME**: An inordinate amount of time spent preparing for, engaging in, and recovering from exercise.

6. **REDUCTION IN OTHER ACTIVITIES**: As a direct result of exercise, social, occupational, and/or recreational activities occur less often or are stopped.

7. **CONTINUANCE**: Continuing to exercise despite knowing that this activity is creating or exacerbating physical, psychological, and/or interpersonal problems.

THE STATISTICS

According to a study from 2013 with 409 men and women:[20]

1. 7.33% of men and women aged 18-22 are exercise dependent.

2. 15.41% of men and women aged 25–44 are exercise dependent.

3. 16.62% of men and women aged 45–64 are exercise dependent.

4. 48% of exercise addicts suffer from eating disorders.

5. 56.3% of exercise addicts suffer from depressive disorders.

6. 46.9% of exercise addicts suffer from personality disorders.

7. 31.3% of exercise addicts suffer from obsessive-compulsive disorders.

THE CAUSES OF EXERCISE ADDICTION

> Self-esteem issues

> Painful life experiences

> Insecurities

> Personality traits like perfectionism, narcissism, and compulsiveness

> Body image issues

> Anxiety

> An addictive personality

> Depression

> A history of eating disorders

> Unrealistic goal setting

> Feelings of not measuring up

People begin exercising for many reasons. They may want to get into better shape, enjoy the program or sport they have decided to participate in or use exercise for stress reduction. Exercise can also be enjoyed in a social setting when done with other people, and for some, it is a safe place where they can take their minds off stressful issues or nagging pain from past events.

Some people will engage in a moderate exercise program and keep the program consistent with only slight modifications when necessary. They are able to maintain a balance in their lives, and exercise is merely one part of that balanced style of life. For others, their exercise program becomes an, and they cannot get enough of it. They think about it when they are not doing it, overdo it when they are, and can become temperamental and angry when they cannot do it. Like any other addiction, compulsive exercise can consume an individual and become something that absolutely must be included in their daily routine, or they may experience withdrawal symptoms like agitation, short temper, and, for some, even physical distress. They will exercise beyond the points of good health, work through pain and injury to keep the program going and put aside responsibilities and significant others as the addiction progresses.

THE SIGNS OF EXERCISE ADDICTION

➤ Feeling guilty or anxious if you do not exercise

➤ Exercising even when it is inconvenient or disruptive to your normal schedule

➤ Thinking about exercise when you are not exercising

➤ Running out of time for other things in your life because you feel you feel that exercise is more important

➤ Feeling withdrawal symptoms when you cannot exercise

➤ Feeling that exercise is not as enjoyable anymore but continuing to exercise anyway.

➤ Exercising even when you have injuries or when you are sick

➤ Skipping work, school, or social events to exercise

➤ Experiencing concerns about physical regression if you cannot workout

THE PROGRESSION

1. The person decides to begin an exercise program. Initially, the exercise may be challenging and uncomfortable.

2. Initially, the exercise may be challenging and uncomfortable.

3. As the person continues, exercise becomes pleasurable, and they develop an exercise program they feel comfortable with.

4. The person begins to experience positive physical gains and feels better emotionally.

5. The person makes slight increases in the program and feels no negative consequences.

6. Feeling more capable, the person increases the frequency and intensity of the workouts.

7. The primary goal starts shifting from enjoyment to challenge, relieving stress and other negative life circumstances, and improving self-esteem and body image.

8. Once again, the frequency and intensity of the program are increased.

9. Realizing the positive gains from the program, exercise becomes a part of the person's life that cannot be missed for any reason.

10. With enhanced concerns about body image and appearance, enjoyment takes a back seat to obsession.

11. The exercise program has become a compulsive act designed to alleviate negative life circumstances and to provide a new, more powerful body image.

12. Self-esteem is now tied directly to the workout program, and the program develops into an exercise addiction.

13. Problems are now beginning to develop as the exercise addict may be experiencing minor injuries and having difficulty organizing their daily schedule around their workout program.

14. When injured, the addict continues to exercise, making whatever modifications in the program are necessary to continue.

15. If the addict cannot exercise, they experience mood swings and irritability.

16. Workouts become considerably longer, and the addict, needing more exercise time, may add additional workouts to their program.

17. The addict adjusts their diet to avoid weight gain as they attempt to achieve the perfect body.

18. The addict has by now become very protective about the exercise program and defends it when challenged by significant others.

19. As the addiction continues, the addict's life revolves around the exercise program. There is less time for family and responsibilities, and their employment may be affected.

20. There is less time for family and responsibilities, and their employment may be affected.

21. Significant amounts of money are being spent on supplements to maximize the workout experience.

22. At this point, the addict is making statements like "I don't know what will happen if I don't work out" and "I can't do without this."

23. The addict now understands that one of the primary reasons to continue at such an extreme pace is to avoid withdrawal since when they stop for several days, they feel uncomfortable and often agitated.

24. Family members are concerned and, at times, angry about the amount of time and persistent dedication spent on the addiction.

25. The addict does not listen to the complaints from family members and rationalizes the behavior as something that is good for their health.

26. The addict sustains an injury or, for some other reason, cannot work out for an extended time and goes into withdrawal.

27. The addict returns to exercising before it is physically safe to do so.

28. The addiction is taking its toll as family relationships are suffering, the addict's health is being negatively affected, their social life is suffering, and their responsibilities have gone unaddressed.

29. Exercise is no longer the addict's "happy place." However, they cannot stop.

Exercise addiction is an example of how something so good can become so bad. The human body is designed for periods of activity followed by periods of rest. Activity should progress to the point that it becomes a bit uncomfortable, and there's nothing wrong with pushing past that point just a bit. However, an exercise addict has no particular limits on how far they are willing to go with their program, nor how much time they spend in it. The human body, especially the muscles, needs time to repair following a strenuous physical workout.

Intense physical exercise breaks the muscles down. The rest period rebuilds them, which is essential in a healthy exercise program. When exercise progresses to the point of addiction, exercise addicts lose their perspective and firmly believe that the more they work out, the stronger they will become. Also, body image, self-esteem, and insecurities attach themselves to the addiction, and without the exercise, the addict may feel as though their world is collapsing around them.

We all need to exercise, but we all need to understand the dynamics of a healthy exercise program and the dangers associated with an exercise obsession that can become unhealthy. When exercise progresses to the point of addiction, the addict becomes unconcerned about negative consequences, compulsively exercising in a desperate attempt to measure up to unattainable goals and to avoid painful withdrawal symptoms.

IN THE CLUTCHES

No addiction is free from the problems and side effects that develop from continued use. What follows is a list of the effects that one can experience from addiction to any drug or activity. Different addictions can lead to different problems, as you will see as we continue.

PHYSICAL PROBLEMS—Exercise addicts often suffer extreme weight loss, joint inflammation, sprained ligaments, dehydration, stress fractures, pressure sores, weakened immune system, chronic exhaustion, sleep issues, failure to fully recover or heal from injuries, illness or other health problems, permanent muscle and joint damage, scarring on the heart muscles, damage to the digestive system due to extreme weight loss, chronic pain, menstrual disturbances and period loss, repeated stress fractures, nerve damage, bone loss, muscle wasting, and adrenal exhaustion.

MENTAL HEALTH ISSUES—Social isolation, depression, anxiety, irritability, mood swings, relationship issues due to obsessive exercise behaviors, becoming fixated on receiving compliments or validation on positive physical changes, basing self-worth on the results of exercise, insecurities, excessive rumination, increases in obsessive-compulsive behaviors, risk of developing eating disorders, risk of developing body image disorders, distorted view of body image or overall well-being, losing close relationships, major depressive disorder, and thoughts of self-harm or suicide are known to plague those addicted to exercise.

COMMUNICATION PROBLEMS—Communication suffers as the addict goes deeper into the addiction, spends more time in the exercise program, is challenged about time spent away from family, and does not take care of their responsibilities. When the addict is not exercising, they may be irritable and temperamental, and communication from the addict can be intense and, at times, abusive.

LEGAL PROBLEMS—The legal problems associated with exercise addiction stem from arrests for using illegal enhancement substances and from violent outbursts that may result from steroid use and other accelerated supplements.

FINANCIAL CONCERNS—Financial concerns are related to excessive purchasing of exercise management products and supplements, work time forfeited to accommodate exercise, buying additional exercise equipment that the addict often cannot afford, and payment for medical expenses when necessary.

FAMILY AND RELATIONSHIP ISSUES—Relationships suffer because the addict is spending excessive amounts of time exercising, they talk about exercising much of the time, and they are angry and reactive when they are in withdrawal. In addition, they spend significant amounts of time away from family members and may miss family outings and events.

EMPLOYMENT PROBLEMS—Employment can suffer because the addict can miss work time both for exercising and because of injury. Also, they cannot be counted on for overtime and other special work projects since these would interfere with their exercise program. At times, they may be reactive at work if they are beginning to feel withdrawal symptoms.

CHANGES IN SOCIAL LIFE—Social life can suffer because the addict will minimize the significance of social interactions and miss social events due to their intense exercise schedule.

LYING—Exercise addicts will lie about how much money they are spending on their addiction, how much time they are going to spend exercising, and the reasons they are not taking care of their responsibilities outside of exercise.

ACCOUNTABILITY ISSUES—Exercise addicts cannot always be counted on since nothing is more important to them than their exercise program. Responsibilities to other people and to their homes often suffer at the hands of the addiction.

PERSONALITY CHANGES—Exercise addicts experience increases in emotional intensity, obsessive-compulsive behavior, and, in the extreme, narcissist behaviors.

ANGER AND VIOLENCE—As the addict becomes stronger and more confident, they may display more aggressive behavior and become over-reactive from taking enhancement supplements. When they experience withdrawal symptoms, they can become angry and, at times, violent.

Certain people are more at risk for exercise addiction. People with eating disorders, body dysmorphic disorder, obsessive-compulsive disorder, ADHD, and those who have personality traits like perfectionism, narcissism, and neuroticism are particularly susceptible. Also, people with past addiction or substance abuse issues, people with a history of addiction within the family, and professional or college athletes are at high risk for this addiction.

COLLATERAL DAMAGE

Though exercise addiction begins as a way to improve one's personal health and physical form, it can quickly develop into an obsessive-compulsive style of living. The addict will start to experience headaches, sleep problems, anxiety and depression, restlessness, loss of appetite, intense feelings of guilt, tension, headaches, and muscle aches. They will also experience periods of withdrawal, which will lead to agitation, exaggerated physical problems, and emotional pain.

The family of an exercise addict, just like all families dealing with addiction, will see their family member's personality change, experience a reduction in the addict's commitment to the family and the home, and experience a drastic decrease in positive interpersonal communication. They will also experience the intensity the exercise addict is living with, their obsession with their body image, their strength, and their need to intensify their program.

While all of this is happening, they will also experience changes in the family dynamics and intimate relationships and the addict's downgrading of priorities that were previously so important to them. As with so many addictions, family members will see themselves as secondary to the addiction, causing them to make decisions that can have a drastic effect on the family. In some cases, those decisions may include leaving the addict.

SUMMING IT UP

It is often difficult to understand the progression from a healthy exercise program to one that can become a serious and detrimental addiction. Exercise stimulates the brain, helps create a stronger body, produces clarity of thought, and settles emotions. While all this is happening, the brain adjusts to the new program, and habit formation sets in. This is where the brain adjusts to the increase in exercise and attempts to accommodate it as it becomes an addiction.

As exercise progresses from a healthy life program to an addiction that can cause pain and severe consequences, it is difficult to pump the brakes and cut back on the intensity of the program. As we have seen with every other addiction, the addict will push past pain and dysfunction and continue to intensify the program. Exercise that becomes an obsession can develop into an addiction. All addictions have that expansive component attached to them; the brain and the body can't seem to get enough of a good thing.

Nothing taken to the extremes is ever positive. Sooner or later, the negative outweighs the positive, and the pain begins. An addictive exercise program can turn a healthy body into one that is broken and painful. While this happens, it has a powerful effect on the entire family. Pay close attention to the progression of this addiction. Be honest with yourself. If you are experiencing an obsessive-compulsive exercise program, help is available. You don't have to stop exercising. You just need to learn how to be healthy about it.

If you or someone you know is addicted to exercise, the addiction hotline is a good place to get help. Call them at (866) 313-2699. Everything is confidential.

 ## TIME TO TAKE ACTION

1. Make an appointment with your primary care physician to ensure that your exercise plan is healthy and not causing any physical problems. Get a blood analysis done. You should do this at least yearly, especially if your exercise program is strenuous.

2. Review the signs and symptoms of exercise addiction listed earlier in the chapter. If you are experiencing these, try to change your program to reduce its impact on you. Start by reducing the amount of time and frequency you work out. If you cannot, it is time to get help.

3. If you are showing signs of exercise addiction, it's a good idea to talk to a personal trainer. You don't have to hire them, but they will give you the correct information to maximize your workouts without them causing problems for you. Hire one if you can.

4. Review your program occasionally with someone who understands the fundamentals of exercise. It is also advisable to talk to a nutritionist to help you avoid taking the wrong supplements and experiencing nutrition-related concerns as your exercise sessions progress.

5. Addiction counselors can help you deal with your exercise addiction. If you cannot stop, there may be underlying reasons, and a counselor can help you address them.

 ## DRIVING IT HOME

Everyone needs some form of exercise to be happy and healthy. That's a fact. Taking exercise too far can turn it into an addiction that can have a drastic impact on the quality of your life. That is also a fact. I have always advised my clients to include an exercise program as part of a healthy living plan. Before you do, schedule a wellness visit with your primary care physician and make sure you are healthy enough to exercise. Before you start exercising, do the research. Understand how to exercise and keep it from becoming problematic in your life. Talk to an exercise professional and get the facts. Use this gift to your advantage, but keep it in perspective. If you do, exercise can be a marvelous, healthy gift that will enhance the quality of your life.

YOUR DECLARATION IS: *I will become knowledgeable about the proper way to exercise, and I will make it a healthy part of my life!*

 ## ONWARD

In the next chapter, I will refer to Chapter 2 of *The Fix Yourself Handbook*. We will explore the necessity of brutal honesty at the beginning of a recovery program. I will discuss how to apply honesty on this level and make it the catalyst for the steps that are necessary to recover from your addiction. **Your blueprint for sober living begins now!**

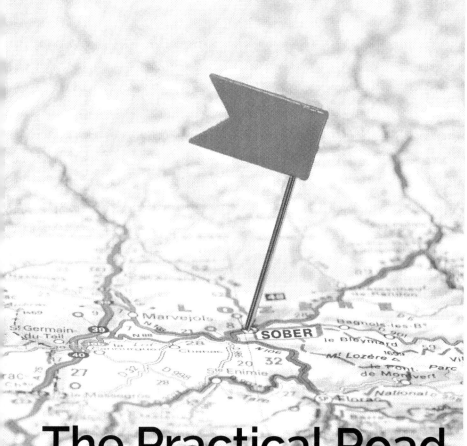

The Practical Road Map to Sobriety: An Opportunity to Fix Your Life

CHAPTER 19

◇◇◇◇◇◇◇◇◇◇◇◇

Getting Honest—
Digging Deep

Honesty tears you down to the core of who you are. Without it, all hope of recovery is gone.

PROCESSES TO EMPLOY: Brutal Honesty, I Over E, Present-Understand-Fix, Slowing Down Life's Pace, Internal Focus, Fact-Finding, Honesty, Patience, Truth-Telling, Belief, Listening, Trust, Humility, Gratitude, Intelligent Decision-Making, Life Inventory

---

I'M GOING TO BE BRUTALLY HONEST WITH you. Addictions are only as strong as the lies and defenses that support them. Addicts live in a world populated both by other addicts and by the "straight" people in their lives. For their addictions to survive, they must con both groups into believing their twisted stories. They can use other addicts to help them maintain their addiction and family and significant others to keep them from compromising it. Addicts need their drugs and their activities of choice. Lies and defenses are the tools these addicted masterminds use to maintain their addictions and to keep potential threats from compromising or bringing to an end what they feel is the most important part of their lives.

In *The Fix Yourself Handbook*, I wrote a chapter titled "Brutal Honesty: The Real Test of Courage." In that chapter, I discuss how everyone claims to be honest and to want honesty from others. However, when they hear the real truth from other people, they can become defensive and quickly go into denial. As this chapter explains, entering an efficient, sustained recovery program is difficult without brutal honesty.

I define "brutal honesty" as *personal truthfulness that is void of defensive thoughts and behaviors and tenaciously seeks the facts, regardless of how they make you feel.* This means you are willing to face the facts, whatever they may be. The facts are the facts, and the facts never change. You must never stop looking for the facts—all of them. You don't want to miss any information that could be crucial to understanding the truth and providing you with that important first step in your recovery.

It is important to dig deep to get the facts. When I teach about brutal honesty, I like to use the analogy of "peeling the onion." The first layer consists of onion paper and the outside skin. There is not much to it, and little of it is usable. It is often discarded. The same applies to the first level of honesty. This layer is filled with emotions, defenses, and sometimes agendas. Most of it is not always useful.

The second layer of the onion makes you feel somewhat uncomfortable, as both your sense of smell and your eyes are affected. So, too, the second level of honesty requires you to go deeper, lose some of the emotions, defenses, and agendas, and work with more of those facts that make you feel uncomfortable.

Then there's that third level, where the real tears begin, and your nose burns just a bit. Now you're uncomfortable. This is where you find brutal honesty. You are uncomfortable because, at this level, you are finally connecting with the truth. There are no defenses, games, or diversions, and your emotions are not controlling your brain. You are facing the facts and only the facts.

THE ADDICT SAYS

If you are an addict, regardless of your drug or activity of choice, manipulation, lies, and misdirection are all mainstays in your addiction toolbox. Addicts are masters of misdirection, diversion, misrepresentation, and twisted tales. The one truth they live by is that they will do anything to maintain the addiction. Almost everything else is lies to keep others off balance and as far away from the truth as possible. Facing the truth means the addict will either admit they have a problem and they are going to do something about it or that they will admit to the problem maliciously because they don't care.

Addicts like to walk that fine line between what they are supposed to do and what they can get away with. This conniving strategy convinces others and themselves that they don't have a problem and that they can stop their addictive behaviors if they choose to do so. They spin ridiculous yarns designed to do nothing more than cover up their addictions and the damage they are causing. They will begin by denying any involvement in the addiction. However, as the addiction continues, they must change their story by either providing a rationale for their actions or attempting to sell their behavior either as insignificant or as a once-in-a-lifetime ordeal.

Once others see through the onion paper misdirection, either they ask more detailed questions or the addict realizes that they are on to them, in which case the addict proceeds to the next level: telling other people that either they have the problem or that the addictive behaviors are the fault of the people accusing them. Initially, family members, loved ones, and significant others will fall for these lies. Soon, however, they will realize they are not the problem, that the addict has been lying to them all along, and that the addiction is continuing to worsen. At the third level of the lie, the addict has become the victim. Now, it's life circumstances, other people's pressures, past pain, and anything else they can conjure up to explain away the addiction.

The most common method of avoiding the brutally honest truth is transferring the blame to other people or situations. The human mind does not like to be attacked and is well-equipped to do what it needs to do to ward off any potential threat. So, addicts blame external forces for their difficulties. This may work for the moment, but it doesn't do anything to help them fix the problem. Consequently, they will continue to repeat the same mistakes.

For an addict to begin the process of recovering from their addiction, they must be brutally honest with themselves. They must be willing to admit that they are wrong and have some flaws and that change needs to occur within them. To make intelligent changes, they must accept the facts in their life with sincere and tenacious truthfulness. If they can do this, they will set the stage for positive change, which leads to sustained personal growth. If you are going to enter a program of recovery from your addiction, it is essential to be a person wearing no masks, one who is completely open and honest. The potential for change, and ultimately growth, starts there.

THE WELL-PEELED ONION

The facts are going to be the facts every day of our lives. Every day, the onion gets peeled. Every day, we face decisions about how truthful we want to be in any situation and whether we will be honest about what is happening. Honesty demands humility, gratitude, consideration for others, and an understanding that the truth is more powerful than the meaningless lies we use to cover it up. The onion of truth, well peeled, dispenses of onion paper misdirection and goes deep to rescue the honesty that can save your life.

There are three basic components of learning to be brutally honest.

1. **THE WILLINGNESS TO PUSH PAST ONION PAPER MISDIREC-TION**—This is the most common level of honesty since it does not challenge you to feel the discomfort that usually accompanies brutal honesty. Brutal honesty requires the willingness to be uncomfortable and still face the facts without their protective lining. It leaves the addict open and vulnerable. That, however, is what truth is. Brutal honesty has no protective devices to shield us from facing truth on truth's terms. If you are serious about starting a recovery program, it is important to understand that it will be uncomfortable but that being completely honest is absolutely necessary.

2. **THE WILLINGNESS TO ACCEPT THE TRUTH WITHOUT DENIAL, PROJECTION, RATIONALIZATION, OR INTELLECTUALIZATION**—For many people, and especially for addicts, truth becomes a product of the defense mechanisms used to alter it. When someone expresses the truth to the addict or the addict is forced to face the truth, they insulate themselves from it using lies and defenses. This creates a half-truth, one that possesses the appearance of honesty but never gets deep enough to face the facts as they exist. This second level of truth

includes a commitment to push past truthless defenses and embrace the facts in any situation. This is where feeling uncomfortable begins.

3. **EMBRACING THE UNCOMFORTABLE FEELINGS THAT COME WITH BRUTAL HONESTY**—Anyone who tells you that you won't feel uncomfortable in the initial stages of getting honest is not being honest with themselves or with you. We use defenses to cover the truth to avoid discomfort and pain. However, being uncomfortable because you are willing to face the facts is the defining measure that tells you that you are being honest. this is where you make the all-important decision to surrender your defenses, lies, and deceit and face the truth about your addiction head-on.

Without the uncomfortable feeling, you are left with defenses, misdirection, and onion paper. Embracing the uncomfortable feelings is where truth begins, and learning takes over. An addict who has decided to be honest with themselves and the rest of the world takes the first step in what can be a sustained recovery program.

When one understands the concept of brutal honesty, accepts it, and incorporates it into one's life, it becomes the most important ally in the fight to stop addiction and begin living a happy, sober life. Almost invariably, addicts who have accepted recovery understand the importance of always being honest with themselves and with everyone else. The moment they begin to lie or misdirect the truth is the moment they can begin to relapse and find themselves right back in the active phase of the addiction.

THE SEVEN KEYS TO HONESTY IN RECOVERY

1. Make it about the facts and only the facts.

2. Listen to your gut. If it feels like a lie, it probably is.

3. Think before you speak. Don't make lying your default response.

4. Always use I over E (intellect over emotion). Think. Feed your brain with factual information.

5. Get uncomfortable. That's where the truth is.

6. Be humble, and don't try to fool or deceive anyone.

7. Be grateful for the truth and make it your best friend.

All addicts lie, and that's the truth. However, those addicts who are truly committed to recovering from their addiction can learn how to be brutally honest. That is also the truth. In Chapter 1, I discussed how one of the brain's primary functions is to keep us happy. Addiction exaggerates the brain's pursuit of pleasure, its defenses, and its pursuit of euphoria. Its defenses will strengthen, and its pursuit of euphoria will continue as the addiction remains active. To help keep the addict satisfied, the brain will abandon the truth. It will lie to its owner and to the rest of the world.

Brutal honesty is the medicine the brain needs to reverse the dishonest, overreactive happiness response that makes it difficult for recovering addicts to separate fact from fiction. Their brains have been subjected to an intense truthless training program, and it will take time to reverse the learning that occurred through this process. Addicts run through stop signs, those warnings that tell them that something is wrong and there could be serious problems. They don't listen to their gut when something feels like a lie. They will have trouble slowing down the default lie response. That's an autopilot behavior, but it is reversible.

Addicts are emotional people. Happiness is felt in the emotional part of the brain, and feeling good is a priority for them. It will take a while for them to understand how to think before they speak so they do not lie and how to apply facts and truthfulness to their responses. Addicts associate discomfort with withdrawal. Their addiction keeps them happy, and withdrawal creates unhappiness. The uncomfortable feeling that often accompanies learning how to be truthful is not easy for an addict to withstand. Humility and addiction have little in common. Addicts are arrogant and use this quasi-strength to keep the addiction going. Admitting they are wrong and being willing to listen to the advice of others is unknown territory, and being grateful for something that makes them uncomfortable and works directly against the addiction seems like a ridiculous premise.

Recovery is hard work. It was never designed to be comfortable, and it is not easy. Some people can come through the addiction, enter recovery, and never look back, but for others, it is quite a different story. The addiction will continue to pull at them. Their brains and emotions will continue searching for quick fixes and immediate gratification, knowing they can find it back in the addiction. To fight the impulse to return to the addiction, the addicts will need all the tools recovery has to offer. The first and most important tool in the recovery toolbox is honesty. It may seem ruthless at times, but honesty can help repair a lifeline spent in turbulent addiction waters.

Honesty is nothing to fear and doesn't always connect one to the more difficult and painful parts of one's life. The brutal honesty I am talking about clears the way to access the beauty deep inside oneself that was hidden by the addiction. It connects to humility and gratitude, attributes that are essential for becoming the powerful person we are all meant to be.

Be willing to face the facts. Be willing to be honest to the point that you are uncomfortable. When you do, you will take the first step in recovering from the physical, emotional, and intellectual slavery caused by the addiction. It will also be the first step to the happy life you have always wanted.

⏱ TIME TO TAKE ACTION

1. Let go of the comfortable and superficial honesty you think you have. Commit to going beyond the way you previously approached honesty. Go deeper and be honest until you feel some discomfort. That's when you know you're arriving at the truth.

2. Try to keep your emotions and defenses to a minimum. The facts are so important now. Don't let your emotions misrepresent them. Don't use old games like denial, intellectualization, and rationalization to misrepresent the truth. Step back and let your brain deal with the facts before your emotions take over.

3. Make being honest all about you. When you feel the urge to lie, ask yourself, "What am I thinking and feeling, and where is this lie coming from?" This will give your brain the time it needs to slow down, examine the facts, and present a more factual representation of what is happening.

4. Try not to be easy on yourself when facing the truth. Go straight to the facts. The facts will show you the best way to become the happy person you want to be.

5. There will be some discomfort as you come to terms with your honest information. This is temporary and necessary if changes are going to be made. Just be as honest with yourself as you can be. Brutal honesty will connect you with parts of yourself you don't like, but change starts there. You *can* do this.

6. Understand that brutal honesty is a life-long process. Don't be afraid of it. If you give it a chance, it will become the best friend you will ever have.

7. Remember this: Addiction is all about lying. Recovery is all about the truth. Whichever of these you choose will define the rest of your life. Choose truth!

 ## DRIVING IT HOME

How honest you are willing to be with yourself will correlate directly to the amount of happiness you will create in your life. Make the commitment to move past your old definition of "honesty," which keeps you comfortable but disconnected from the accurate information you need as you begin the initial stages of your recovery. Be willing to accept a bit of discomfort. Discomfort tells you that you're growing. The facts will always be the facts. Learn to love them. Doing so can make the truth one of your most important recovery allies.

YOUR DECLARATION IS: *I will face the facts, get uncomfortable, learn about myself, and live a happy and productive life!*

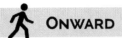 ONWARD

In the next chapter, I will take an in-depth look at the games addicts play even as they enter the initial stages of recovery. I will look at how defenses apply at this stage and how addicts attempt to manipulate others while also fooling themselves into believing that this stage of the recovery process is permanent.

◇◇◇◇◇◇◇◇◇◇◇◇

CHAPTER 20

Giving Up the Games— Saying Goodbye to Manipulation

It is the powerful white flag. It says I am done with this life, and I am done fighting myself.

PROCESSES TO EMPLOY: Brutal Honesty, I Over E, Present-Understand-Fix, Slowing Down Life's Pace, Internal Focus, Fact-Finding, Honesty, Patience, Truth-Telling, Belief, Listening, Trust, Intelligent Decision-Making, Life Inventory, Conflict Resolution, Language Reciprocity

---

I DEFINE "ADDICTION RECOVERY" as *a process of change through which individuals improve their health and wellness, live a self-directed life, and strive to reach their full potential.* Examining this definition, we find three distinct components:

1. **IMPROVING HEALTH AND WELLNESS**—This refers to the addict's physical, emotional, intellectual, and spiritual health. Recovery programs, especially 12-step programs, tend to focus on all four attributes.

2. **LIVING A SELF-DIRECTED LIFE**—Regardless of the drug or activity an addict engages in, it can take over their lives and direct the course of them. Recovery programs strive to teach addicts how to direct their own lives efficiently and compassionately with the drug or addictive activity.

3. **STRIVING TO REACH ONE'S FULL POTENTIAL**—By living a balanced life free from addiction, recovering addicts can learn to identify their talents and use them to reach their maximum potential.

Living this kind of life is the antithesis of the one the addict is used to living. It requires learning new skills and taking the advice of others. It also requires hard work, a willingness to take the advice of others who understand recovery, and focusing on improving all aspects of health and wellness without compromise. Addicts aren't big fans of hard work, and the whole concept of "sobriety for the long haul" seems a bit sketchy. So, the addict's initial version of sobriety isn't so accepting of the "without compromise" component as they like to include a little more wiggle room, a touch of bargaining, and as much self-centered compromise as possible in their plan.

One of the most fundamental concepts for a new recovering addict to understand is that they are no longer in control of the program. This is a hard pill for an addict to swallow. Although an addict's life operates out of control, they have to control everyone and everything they can to protect their addiction. Now, they are suddenly being asked to relinquish control, to embrace the big picture for the long haul, to be honest, and to work hard. These concepts have almost no place in an addict's previous lifestyle.

NOT SUCH A CLEAR PATH

Before an addict grasps the principles of recovery, they attempt to stop using without training their brain to make the change from an addicted lifestyle to one of sobriety. They don't have a full understanding of what sobriety is, what it takes to begin the process, and what it takes to maintain it. There is a dysfunctional marriage between the initial decision to try sobriety and trying to do so with a mind that is not prepared to understand the concept. This is one of the reasons why any good program of sobriety moves slowly, taking a step-by-step approach, always under the guidance of a professional and a support team.

Until addicts begin to understand the process and are willing to surrender their will to those who know more about sober living, they will attempt to incorporate items in their old toolbox into their new way of living. They will enter a recovery program while trying to be comfortable in the process. This typically amounts to trying to adjust to recovery using some of the strategies they used in the addiction. This is what it looks like:

- ➤ **BARGAINING**—Instead of taking advice as it is given and attempting to do the work suggested by others who are more knowledgeable about recovery, they will attempt to make some improvements while trying to negotiate the parts that require more effort.

- ➤ **HALF-TRUTHS**—Instead of being completely honest, they give some of the facts and tell selected parts of a story as they attempt to maintain control in a program that demands surrender. They are masters at the art of providing partial truths.

- ➤ **PARTIAL COOPERATION**—They will view partial cooperation as considerably better than how they used to behave, thinking that some cooperation is better than none and should be appreciated by those advising them.

- ➤ **VICTIMIZATION**—When they become uncomfortable and others urge them to do more work, they may suggest that this is unfair and that others are taking advantage of them.

- ➤ **PASSIVE-AGGRESSIVE BEHAVIOR**—At times, though they want to convince those helping them that they are trying to do the right thing, they will sabotage the program to do less work. For example, they may schedule a conflicting appointment to avoid a recovery-focused commitment or pretend to be sick to avoid responsibility.

- ➤ **CLAIMING TO BE MISUNDERSTOOD**—When they are urged to do more work and can't see a way out of it, they will accuse others of not understanding who they are and how much effort it takes to do the difficult tasks being demanded.

- ➤ **PROCRASTINATION**—They will continue to avoid their responsibilities and must be reminded to get things done.

- ➤ **DOING THINGS HALFWAY**—They will start tasks without completing them, maybe doing just enough to get by.

- ➤ **MISDIRECTION**—They will continue to try to misdirect people by diverting attention away from the task at hand and to some other more difficult situation, at least as they see it.

- ➤ **MANIPULATION**—They will do their best to try to convince others that there are better ways to do what they are being asked, and they will perform other, more simple tasks to convince others that they are invested in the program.

Some addicts fake recovery because they have received ultimatums from those who care about them and don't want to lose what they still have. Others may be involved in court actions and have been mandated into a recovery program. Some may have lost a great deal in their lives and are sincere about attempting to leave the addiction behind. Those who receive ultimatums or are mandated into treatment will use games and manipulation to convince others that they are trying when they have no intention of investing themselves in the program, while those who are making a sincere effort may still use their old tricks as they attempt to understand how to live without them.

"FAKE IT TILL YOU MAKE IT" DEBUNKED

Recovery from any addiction is an all-or-nothing proposition. There is no halfway, no leeway, and no faking it until you make it. All of these lead to temptation since anything short of a total commitment includes menacing addiction residue. Addiction residue is the intellectual and sometimes physical craving that pulls you back into the active phase of the addiction. If the addict isn't fully committed to the recovery plan, the brain and the body become caught between the halfhearted attempt at recovery and the obsessive chase after the euphoria attached to the addiction. This creates an internal war that can result in disaster for the addict.

In the initial stages of recovery, no addict knows what they are getting themselves into. Typically, they know what they don't want: They don't want the pain and loss associated with addiction. They don't want to hurt family members anymore. They don't want to hurt their bodies and their minds, and they don't want to be emotional wrecks. Many addicts have expressed how nice it would be to be able to indulge in their drug of choice without experiencing all the pain and loss associated with the addiction. It is difficult to leave something that may have produced some of your life's most euphoric and enjoyable experiences, even though it took so much of your life away from you.

In recovery, there can be no halfway. There are no cheat days, no once-in-a-whiles, no maybes, and definitely no trying to talk other people into an easier way of making sobriety and the work associated with it easier to implement. Attempting to incorporate any of these compromises into a program of sobriety does nothing more than sabotage the program and lead directly back to the addiction. There is no compromise in sobriety. Negotiating and attempting to convince others to do it your way doesn't work. You wouldn't need a recovery program if you could do it your way. Your way, however, is what got you into this mess. It certainly isn't going to get you out of it.

THE CLEARER PATH

Earlier in this chapter, I discussed how addicts try to adjust to recovery using some of the strategies they used in the addiction. These strategies cannot work in recovery. Let's take a look at the adjustments the addict needs to make to keep every one of these strategies from sabotaging their recovery. I will present this as advice being delivered specifically to the addicts. This is what it looks like:

➤ **BARGAINING**—Before an addict attempts to bargain with others, they have decided upon and rehearsed the bargaining language with themselves. Stopping this internal dialogue before it becomes an overt delivery is the first step to stopping the bargaining process. As soon as you begin the internal conversation, recognize it for the red flag it is and stop it. If you do, you are less likely to try bargaining with the people who are trying to help you.

➤ **HALF-TRUTHS**—Recovery is an all-or-nothing proposition. If you alter part of the story or leave some important details out, you deal with half-truths. This is a deliberate strategy unless you are a compulsive liar who cannot separate facts from fiction. To avoid this, present the entire story with all the facts all the time.

➤ **PARTIAL COOPERATION**—Partial cooperation is not cooperation at all. It is doing just enough to get by. Recovery requires a total commitment. It demands your cooperation in full, always. This doesn't mean you have to be perfect. It simply means you must try your best in every situation and with everyone in your life.

➤ **VICTIMIZATION**—There are only victims in addiction; there are no victims in recovery. Using victimization to get others to pity you so they can make things easy for you is a self-imposed attack on your dignity and your humanity. Leave your victimization in the addiction. Don't feel sorry for yourself because you have decided to change your life. It's time to rise to the occasion.

➤ **PASSIVE-AGGRESSIVE BEHAVIOR**—Being passive-aggressive is an old addiction tool, a defense used to cover up anger. In recovery, anger is nothing more than something to be worked on, and it's one of the personality flaws that kept the addiction alive. It makes no sense to attempt to hurt the people helping you. If you are contemplating ways to punish those people who are committing themselves to your recovery program, you are sabotaging yourself. If you are purposefully hurting someone, apologize quickly and return to the work you need to do to help yourself.

➤ **CLAIMING TO BE MISUNDERSTOOD**—No one will always understand you. If you feel you're being misunderstood, try to have a positive conversation with the other person and make your feelings known, but do this with the understanding that it will not get you out of the work that sobriety demands. The only reason to discuss this issue is to help someone understand who you are so they can help you more efficiently, not so they will go easier on you. That is not their job, and your job is to embrace your sobriety and all the hard work that goes along with it.

- ➤ **PROCRASTINATION**—Procrastination is deciding when, how, and how much you want to give to recovery and making it known to yourself and those supporting you that you are unwilling to embrace it all. Nothing about sobriety works that way. Every day is new; every day has things that need to be done and done in a timely fashion. The longer you put off recovery, the longer it will take to get well, and the more likely you are to return to the addiction. Do it now.

- ➤ **DOING THINGS HALFWAY**—As stated in this chapter, there is no such thing as halfway in recovery. You have people advising and supporting you, helping you create a path to a healthier and more productive way of life. They are not giving you half-truths or half the advice you need to succeed. Don't give yourself or them half an effort. Be willing to put your best foot forward all the time.

- ➤ **MISDIRECTION**—Remember that when you attempt to misdirect others so you don't have to do the work, you are misdirecting yourself. If these others are already sober and living a sober life, they're reaping the rewards of their work. You're not going to fool them into believing your misdirections. Stay on point, follow the directions, and do what you must.

- ➤ **MANIPULATION**—Keep in mind that most of the people helping you, particularly people like counselors, sponsors, and other sober people, understand the addiction game; they will see your manipulations long before you acknowledge them to yourself. Attempting to manipulate those who already know better amounts to nothing but making a fool of yourself. Be straight with them and with yourself, and stop trying to control the world.

This is your life you are trying to save. You're not going to do so by doing things halfway or by playing the old games you used to use in addiction. One of the most important facts that addicts tend to miss is that although other people care about them and desperately want them to succeed, they have no control over the addict, they cannot be susceptible to their games, and they will not allow the addict's games to have a negative impact on their lives.

If you successfully use your old games and manipulate the people trying to help you, you won't beat them. You'll beat yourself. When you look back, this is exactly what happened in the addiction. You may have routinely conned everyone else into believing your lies, but in the end, it was your life that was seriously affected. If you attempt to use your old games in your new program, it will only take you back to where you were in the addiction. Those around you who are working hard will continue to embrace their sobriety program. The decision to relinquish your old tricks and embrace a way of life that can restore your health and your family is entirely up to you to make.

 TIME TO TAKE ACTION

1. Let others guide you as you enter the initial stages of your recovery. They will go slow, and nothing they advise will be impossible for you to accomplish.

2. Pay close attention to the sections entitled "Not Such a Clear Path" and "The Clearer Path" in this chapter. Study them. The first one lists the old tools you used in addiction and how they can work against you. The second tells you how to reverse the process with each of them. Follow the advice in these sections.

3. You can't do this alone. Since addiction often has underlying pain and trauma associated with it, it's a good idea to have someone to talk to. There are addiction counselors who can help you. Your primary care physician may help you identify a counselor who can help you, or you can go online to find one. Psychology Today is a good source for finding addiction counselors. Make an appointment with one of them.

4. Support programs such as AA, NA, Gamblers Anonymous, etc., are available to help you with your addiction. You can find support programs to help you with the type of addiction you are addressing online. Attend one of their meetings. Some are held in physical

meeting rooms, while others can be attended in virtual formats. You will learn a lot there, and you can develop an invaluable network of people who can help you with your recovery.

 ## DRIVING IT HOME

Your addiction was your own, but if you try to make your recovery your own, prepare to return to the ways you followed in addiction because those are the only ways you know. That's why you fell so deep into the addiction. Your sobriety, in large part, will be based upon the knowledge, experience, and wisdom of those guiding you. They have been in the trenches; they understand the addiction and what you were doing to maintain it, and they know the way out. The formula to get started is simple: Leave your arrogance at the door, embrace humility, and listen to those who know more than you do. If you do, it just might save your life.

YOUR DECLARATION IS: *I will be humble and let others be the guiding light in my new life!*

 ## ONWARD

In the next chapter, I will examine addiction substitutes. Though they may not be the addiction of choice, these are substitutes that keep the addictive state of mind operative and introduce setups that pave the way for program relapses.

CHAPTER 21

◇◇◇◇◇◇◇◇◇◇◇◇◇

Addiction Substitutes—
Replacement Wastelands

Forget the replacements. They are nothing more than an extension of an addictive style of life. Embrace sobriety and quit the quick fixes.

PROCESSES TO EMPLOY: Brutal Honesty, I Over E, Present-Understand-Fix, Slowing Down Life's Pace, Internal Focus, Fact-Finding, Honesty, Slowing Down Life's Pace, Internal Focus, Patience, Truth-Telling, Belief, Listening, Trust, Intelligent Decision-Making, Life Inventory, Conflict Resolution, Reduction of Destination Living

---

IN CHAPTER 2, I INTRODUCED THE NOTION that the addict can suffer from more than one addiction at a time. It is not uncommon for a person with an addictive personality to find themselves drawn into several addictive substances or activities, usually preferring one as their addiction of choice. In this chapter, I will take a deeper look at what happens when a person begins a recovery program, only to find themselves switching addictions and convincing themselves that no longer being involved in the primary addiction despite switching to another compulsive behavior at the same time is acceptable in a recovery program.

An example of a replacement addiction is stopping drinking but indulging in late-night comfort eating, resulting in excessive weight gain. Another example is stopping the use of methamphetamine but increasing caffeine intake. It's one thing to stop using one's addiction of choice;

however, indulging in a new addiction is nothing more than remaining in addiction. Switching addictions is problematic for two reasons:

1. It keeps the addict's addictive personality engaged in an obsessive-compulsive routine.

2. Since the addictive personality remains engaged, it increases the likelihood that the person will become addicted to a different substance or behavior, or they may even return to the original addiction.

An important function of the human brain is to keep its owner happy and comfortable. Addicts don't like to be uncomfortable; it makes them unhappy. Finding a replacement addiction, though it is not always a conscious decision, is a shrewd way to keep that addictive brain overproducing neurotransmitters as it reestablishes the euphoric world that is so important to the addict. An addict who switches their addiction to another substance or activity can tell themselves and the rest of the world that they are in recovery. This is one of those half-truths. They may have stopped engaging in the original addictive activity, but they are still actively addicted. Let's take a look at an example of this process:

Bonnie is a thirty-seven-year-old dental assistant. She is divorced and has no children. She comes from a family of alcoholics, though all of them were "functional drinkers"; they all went to work and cared for their homes and families, and their responsibilities were routinely addressed. However, most of them drank every evening, often to excess, and were intoxicated for the better part of the weekend.

Bonnie's drinking pattern mirrors that of her parents: Bonnie goes to work every day, is efficient on the job, and is well respected by her employers, for whom she has worked for fourteen years. She is active in the community and cares for her home and two dogs. After she takes care of her responsibilities following her workday, she settles in, watches television, and typically drinks four or five large glasses of wine. However, she gets up every morning and returns to work and her responsibilities.

Three months ago, after drinking, Bonnie ran a quick errand to the corner store. On the way back, she swerved to avoid hitting a cat, hit the curb, and got a flat tire. A local police officer stopped to assist her and smelled the alcohol on her breath. Bonnie was arrested for a DUI. During her court-ordered evaluation, she scored high on the addiction scale and, for the first time, admitted that she has a problem. Part of her court-ordered alcohol program was to attend a group counseling program. She liked the counselor running the group and scheduled an appointment with her to address her alcohol consumption and a few other personal concerns.

The counselor was an addiction specialist, and Bonnie understood that she not only had a problem with alcohol but that she was, in fact, an alcoholic. Bonnie decided to stay with the counselor and attended her first AA meeting with a friend who was a recovering alcoholic. Bonnie decided that she was going to quit drinking, keep going to counseling, and attend at least one meeting per week. After two months, Bonnie has not consumed alcohol, but something else happened.

Since Bonnie saved approximately $50 a week on alcohol, she decided that she would spend $5 at the local convenience store and purchase a lottery ticket. As fate would have it, Bonnie won $25 on her first ticket. Bonnie decided to use that $25 to purchase five more tickets. One of those tickets was a winning ticket. Bonnie enjoyed her low-stakes games of chance and decided to move up to the weekly lottery; the purse was big, and Bonnie was already thinking about what she would do with the money if she won.

The numbers were announced, and Bonnie didn't win, but she found herself looking forward to next week's drawing. She began talking about her new hobby with patients who came into the office, and one woman invited her to go to the casino with her. Bonnie obliged and loved the experience.

Bonnie now goes to the casino on Saturday and Sunday afternoons. Bonnie has begun a gambling addiction.

TRADING PLACES

If you look at recovery as the successful movement away from a primary addiction, Bonnie is a recovering alcoholic. Unfortunately, she is also now an active gambling addict. She has traded one addiction for another.

In her alcohol addiction, Bonnie was spending $50 a week and getting drunk in the evenings. She was going to work, took care of her responsibilities at home, and was active in the community.

In her new addiction, she continued to go to work and excel there. She came home at the end of the day, took care of her responsibilities, watched television, and began to read a little more than she used to. Not much has changed, except that Bonnie's financial commitment to her new addiction is about four times more than she had been spending on alcohol. In addition, Bonnie has to travel just under 25 miles, round trip, to the casino. Bonnie feels the euphoria that gambling provides her and, in her mind, gives herself a little pat on the back that she is no longer drinking.

However, referring back to the potential problems when one uses a replacement addiction, Bonnie is still an active addict; she is just addicted to something else. In addition, Bonnie is gambling in a place where alcohol flows freely. For now, she isn't paying attention to the alcohol. However, the likelihood of that addiction returning is significantly increased because she is still actively addicted to something else and engaging in that new addiction in a place that serves alcohol.

I have discussed how manipulative addicts can be, and I have also discussed how efficiently the brain works in helping the addict maintain the addiction. I have also talked about how when addicts trick other people, they are often also tricking themselves. In the case of addiction replacements, the addict may know that the new behavior is an addiction and that it is harmful. However, at times, that efficient thinking machine, without its owner's understanding of what it's doing, can make a quick substitution to keep the euphoric experience alive.

Addiction substitutes are not always a conscious choice by the addict. It's important to understand that an addictive personality doesn't have to be something the addict consciously understands or consciously thinks about. It is often an unconscious, autopilot way of living. It is life du jour. It is the default normal way of living for an addict. So, the jump from one addiction to another is not only something that can be unconscious but can also be seamless. It's one of those behaviors that can be difficult to identify until one is knee-deep in it.

BRAIN ENGAGED

The addict must be aware of the possibility of switching to another addiction from the moment they decide to enter into recovery. Recovery is not a destination; it's a lifelong journey. One does not simply stop the primary addiction, and all addiction ends there. The primary addiction was the initial expression of the addictive personality, but it was not the final expression. The reason addicts will say they will always be addicts is that the addictive personality doesn't simply pack up and leave. It's the part of the addict that is always available and can always attach itself to a new drug or a new activity.

Understanding the addictive personality and the possibility of it attaching to several different drugs or activities during the active phase of the addiction is crucial to recovery. Being aware of this possibility can help an addict and their treatment team plan an efficient recovery program. Addiction counselors and 12-step programs routinely teach the concept of staying away from other addictive people, places, and things because they understand how easy it is to move from one addiction to another. The best way to start a recovery program is to understand that the addictive personality will always be there and can attach to other addictive devices and to include that knowledge in your recovery program.

1. 7 Keys to Avoiding Addiction SubstitutesLearn as much as you can about the addictive personality.

2. Avoid high-risk people, places, and things.

3. Include a counselor and support people in your recovery plan.

4. The urge to do anything that could develop into an addiction can threaten your sobriety. Discuss it with your counselor, sponsor, or other support people.

5. Report any changes or new behaviors to those helping you as soon as they begin, even if they seem insignificant.

6. If you become involved in an addictive substance or behavior, talk to your counselor or support team immediately.

7. If you start using an addictive substitute, include the recovery from that drug or behavior in your recovery plan alongside your primary addiction.

The most important takeaway from this chapter is that although the primary goal is to stop using your current drug or activity of choice, it is also important to recognize that being an addict means you have an addictive personality. This personality attaches itself to one drug or activity and can just as efficiently attach itself to another. Addicts must keep this addictive potential in mind as they enter recovery to mitigate the possibility of transferring the addiction to another drug or activity.

The best way to deal with addiction is to remove yourself from anything that can be addictive. That's easier said than done. The addiction will always be calling your number. That's why addiction recovery programs are lifelong programs. It is commendable to stop using your primary drug or activity, and you should feel good about that. Just remember that while you are focusing on that life-threatening demon, another smaller one may sneak up right behind it.

TIME TO TAKE ACTION

1. Your first step is to address your primary addiction. Focus on that one first. Follow the advice of those who are helping you, and be honest with them.

2. Involve yourself with an addiction counselor and a 12-step program. This will help you to address your personal concerns and provide the support you need to help you with your addictive personality.

3. Learn everything you can about the addictive personality. Your sponsor and support team can help you acquire and understand this information. There is also a wealth of information on this subject online.

4. Pay attention to the 7 Keys to Avoiding Addiction Substitutes. Share them with your counselor and your sponsor or support team. This will help you include them as part of your addiction recovery plan.

5. Report any thoughts and activities about potentially addictive substances or activities to your counselor and support team. It's so important to address these issues as early as possible.

 DRIVING IT HOME

Addictive personalities attach themselves to addictive substances and activities. Constructing an efficient recovery program means addressing the primary addiction and any other addictions that may ride on its coattails. It is so important to keep your focus on your addictive personality, your primary addiction, and any others that may enter life. Addressing the primary addiction must come first since it has the potential to be serious enough to take your life. Do that first, but never forget that an addict remains an addict always. You can relapse back to your primary addiction, or you can replace it with another drug or activity. The question is whether you want to be an active addict or a recovering addict. Think about this one carefully.

YOUR DECLARATION IS: *I will keep my mind focused on my addictive personality and the lifelong plan I must use to address it!*

 ONWARD

In the next chapter, I will examine the difference between positive and negative family and peer associations. I will pay special attention to how positive influencers can help you rise above addictive turmoil and how negative influencers can drive you back to addiction.

◇◇◇◇◇◇◇◇◇◇◇◇◇

CHAPTER 22

People, Places, and Things— Saviors or Setups

We live and die by the choices we make. Who, where, and what we choose can be our saving graces or our life-destroying demons.

PROCESSES TO EMPLOY: Brutal Honesty, I Over E, Present-Understand-Fix, Slowing Down Life's Pace, Internal Focus, Fact-Finding, Honesty, Patience, Truth-Telling, Belief, Listening, Trust, Intelligent Decision-Making, Life Inventory, Conflict Resolution, Reduction of Destination Living, Goal Setting, Living in the Moment, One-Day-at-a-Time Living, Boundary-Setting

---

MANY YEARS AGO, ALCOHOLICS ANONYMOUS began telling those in recovery from alcoholism that they should understand the potential dangers involved in associating with negative people, places, and things. To maintain sobriety, recovering alcoholics are urged to avoid any person, place, or thing that might compromise their sobriety. In *The Fix Your Anxiety Handbook*, I wrote a chapter about including the right people, places, and things in your life to help you work through anxiety. Some of that material is included in this chapter because the same good advice applies to your recovery from whatever addiction you are up against.

We all live and die as a result of the choices we make. The people you include in your life can significantly affect how you think, feel, and behave. I define "people, places, and things" as *those individuals, locations, objects, activities, and events that enter your life and can have a positive, negative, or neutral effect on you.*

I have discussed habit formation at length and how, by repeating thoughts and behaviors over time, your brain adjusts to accommodate these thoughts and behaviors. In yet another version of this normalizing process, your brain can adapt to experiences with the people, places, and things involved in your life. This is significant because, as I have discussed, what you choose to include in your life can either help you create positive energy to move you forward or have negative implications. Rarely do the people, places, or things you allow to enter your life do so without affecting you.

By reading this book, you are trying to create positive energy, which will help you remove addiction from your life and create a lifestyle that supports healthy functioning. Anything that affects how your body generates and uses energy is important. The people you associate with, the places you frequent, the things you do, and even the objects you own all affect your ability to create and use energy. All can gain permanence in your life if they remain in your life long enough.

THE PEOPLE

The people you choose to associate and interact with can influence the way you live. Positive people help bring positive energy into your life. Their qualities should include:

- Loyalty
- Trustworthiness
- Supportiveness
- Willingness to listen
- Emotional availability
- Unconditional acceptance
- Honesty
- Helpfulness
- Kindness
- Love
- Genuineness
- Dependability

There are also those people who can bring negative energy into your life. Such people can be:

- Untrustworthy
- Judgmental
- Undependable
- Often distant

- Selfish
- Gossips
- Possessive
- Exploitative
- Disloyal; they may betray you
- Critical
- Frequently untruthful

Humans are social animals. Depending on your personal needs, your positive relationships can range from mildly warm and supportive to essential. Considering your need for that all-important human touch and all the qualities a good friend can bring into your life, the people you allow to get close to you can significantly impact the quality of your life.

Good friends should feed your intellect. In a supportive fashion, they should challenge you, present you with information that helps you expand your intellectual database, and, at times, assume the role of a good teacher. As I stated previously, teaching and learning can occur in various venues. A good friend can also learn from you and should value your opinions.

Emotionally, good friends let you know that you are important to them. They make you feel safe, loved, and accepted, regardless of those little flaws and imperfections that everyone has. They will go the extra mile for you if you need them. You never feel like you are a burden to them, and you feel that they look forward to seeing you. You can laugh or cry with them, and they make you feel accepted and appreciated.

Good friends can also significantly impact you physically. You can enjoy a nice hug with them and you can also enjoy including them in your personal physical space. There's also that mind-to-body connection, which I have discussed in the other books in The Fix Yourself Empowerment Series. As you feel the positive energy, intellectually and emotionally, coming from the supportive people in your life, it has a calming effect on your body.

THE PLACES

I define "places" as *a space available or designated for use by someone.* The places you choose to include in your life should be physically, intellectually, and emotionally safe. There should be no threat of violence, and you should feel comfortable there. A positive place should reinforce your quest for peace and your desire for ongoing personal growth. These places should not bring negative energy into your life.

Alcoholics Anonymous tells us that a safe place for a recovering person is one that does not challenge their sobriety. This being the case, it might not be a good idea for a recovering alcoholic to visit a bar or attend a party where large amounts of alcohol are served. The temptation in either venue could be great, and the possibility of slipping back into old, negative ways of thinking and behaving would increase.

When it comes to sobriety, avoid places that increase negative thinking and those that feed the addiction. Sometimes, this may require you to physically leave a triggering venue. Other times, the place might be right inside your own mind. For example, spending time at a not-so-positive friend's house might trigger old negative thoughts, or how they talk and behave might cause your mind and emotions to regress back to old negative thoughts and behaviors. It would be a good idea to avoid spending time in such a place.

When it comes to your mind, it doesn't have to be brick-and-mortar changes that can cause you to regress. Think of your mind as composed of many different places you can visit, intellectually and emotionally. It is important to avoid these demon-feeding spaces such as a bar room, the casino, or a dysfunctional relationship. Keep your mind focused on positive places, those that don't challenge your sobriety, and enhance your program of recovery.

Safe places are, among other things:

➤ Free of physical danger

➤ Emotionally stable

➤ Free of temptation

➤ Full of positive energy

➤ Supportive of personal growth

➤ A venue for positive people

➤ Supportive of positive thinking and behaviors

➤ Intellectually stimulating

➤ Havens of peace and tranquility

The places you choose to frequent can have a significant impact on your growth and your movement away from the addiction. There are two rules to abide by 1) Avoid the places you know could cause a rise in negative energy or put you in danger physically, intellectually, or emotionally, and 2) If you find yourself in a place that feels as though it may bring on negative energy, remove yourself from that place as fast as you can. Keeping your life places safe and positive goes a long way toward ridding yourself of the addiction's influence and finding the happiness that is so important to you.

THE THINGS

We all have things that are important to us or that make us feel good. Some things can make you feel better than you otherwise would; others can even add a new and exciting dimension to your life. When you like something, as I have discussed, you tend to continue to include it in your life. Repeating the experience is comforting, and the pleasure you feel makes you look forward to doing the same thing again.

As I define it, "things" are *the objects and experiences you may add to your life, either because you have become accustomed to doing so or because you believe that they increase the quality of your life in some manner.* Some of those things enhance your quality of life. They may include:

- Reading a good book
- Your Bible
- Your treadmill
- Your music
- Listening to a podcast about good nutrition
- A mat that you use to practice yoga
- Automobiles and other "toys"

You may include these things in your life that can create or enhance positive energy flow.

However, some things you choose to include in your life can cause problems for you. Examples of those things might include:

- Substance abuse
- Mementoes that cause you to ruminate over painful past experiences
- Comfort foods that can cause physical problems

- Objects, insignias, and other items that represent anger and violence

- Negative forms of social media

Life is full of things with both positive and negative energy attached to them. Assess the effect the things you include in your life have on you. If they cause you to feel negative, fearful, angry or make you feel bad about yourself, it may be a good idea to rid yourself of them. If they create potentially problematic comfort zones, it's advisable to avoid them. Also, if you become obsessive about them, and this causes you to ruminate or revisit past pain, it's better to part with them. Consider anything with a negative charge to be powerful enough to lead you back to the addiction—something to be avoided at all costs. Try to include only things that add something positive to your life.

KEEP IT IN PERSPECTIVE

Pay attention to the potential effects the people, places, and things you include in your life have on you. Ask yourself these two simple questions: "Will including this in my life help create positive energy to help me become happier and more productive? Is there any danger of returning to the addiction, or could there be some collateral damage if I choose to include this in my life?"

Remember, the addiction thrives on negativity and pain. Everything you are doing, as I am outlining it, is designed to weaken and eventually cast out the beast. People, places, and things will always be part of your life and can add that wonderful new dimension that leads to the happiness and productivity you seek. Understanding how to incorporate them into your life is yet one more powerful weapon in your fight against addiction.

TIME TO TAKE ACTION

1. Make a list of all the people you associate with. Divide that list into two: one of the people who support your sobriety and one of those who threaten that sobriety.

2. Make a second list of all the places you visit in your attempt to maintain a healthy lifestyle. Again, break that list down into places that support your continued recovery from your addiction and those that have the potential to return you to your addictive lifestyle.

3. Make a third list of everything you do or have in your life. This may include negative mementos, comfort foods, pornographic videos, and over-the-counter substances that change the way you feel, to list a few. Break this list down into those things and events that are healthy and keep you focused on an addiction-free lifestyle and those that may cause you to return to the grasp of the addiction.

4. With these lists made and separated, formulate a plan that helps you avoid the problematic people, places, and things and enhances your recovery from your addiction and your movement into a healthy, sober life. Share this list with your counselor or support people to help you discern who/what stays and who/what goes.

 ## DRIVING IT HOME

Become willing to consciously evaluate who and what you include in your life and who and what you choose to exclude. Learn to become your own personal gatekeeper. Surround yourself with people who are positive and healthy. Choose to go to places and events that support your recovery and your personal health. Include things and events that facilitate the healthy lifestyle you have chosen to embrace. This is your life we're talking about. Become the master of your own destiny.

Choose carefully who and what gets in, and keep anything and anyone who threatens your health and your sobriety from entering your life.

YOUR DECLARATION IS: *I will include only those people, places, and things in my life that help me maintain my sobriety and my happiness!*

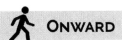 **ONWARD**

Almost every addict has family members who have been on the addiction roller coaster with them. In the next chapter, I will examine how important the recovery process is, not only for the addict but also for their family and other loved ones. I will look at what family members need to do to support the addict with their sobriety, but also to ensure they obtain the help they need to become healthy.

CHAPTER 23

It's a Family Affair:
We Are All Connected

It has a way of biting into everyone. No addiction occurs in a void.

PROCESSES TO EMPLOY: Brutal Honesty, I Over E, Present-Understand-Fix, Slowing Down Life's Pace, Internal Focus, Fact-Finding, Honesty, Slowing Down Life's Pace, Internal Focus, Patience, Truth-Telling, Belief, Listening, Trust, Intelligent Decision-Making, Life Inventory, Conflict Resolution, Reduction of Destination Living, Goal Setting, Living in the Moment, One-Day-at-a-Time Living, Boundary-Setting, Warm Communication, Settling Past Issues

---

ALMOST EVERYTHING WE DO TOUCHES THOSE CLOSE TO US. We like to assume that since we are the owners of our own lives, we have the right to live any way we choose and do anything we choose. We also like to assume that our choices do not impact others.

In this fast-paced, technological world, we often discuss the concept of connectivity. No form of connectivity is more deep-reaching than the connection between family members. What one does always affects one's family. Whether it is winning the lottery or going bankrupt, whether it is good health or some horrible disease, whether one is laid back and supportive or angry and temperamental, it all has its effect on those we live with. Addiction is no exception to the rule.

Addiction's impact on the family is often intense, deep-reaching, and life-changing. The addict is not the only person held tight in the grasp of this unrelenting slave master. Those who live with, work with, are in relationships with, and even socialize with the addict will experience, in one way or another, the pain of the addiction.

COLLATERAL DAMAGE EXPANDED

In chapters 3 through 18, I discussed collateral damage—that is, the damage to family and friends caused by addiction. As you saw in those chapters, each addiction has its own progression—its own way of wrapping its clutches around people—and each addiction also carries the potential for significant collateral damage. "Collateral damage" is typically defined as *any incidental and undesired death, injury, or other damage inflicted on those who are not part of the original action.* When one decides to do something dangerous, the possibility of inflicting death or injury on another person cannot be ignored.

Collateral damage as it relates to addiction is caused by the power of the addiction and, subsequently, the addict's poor decisions. This can have a dramatic impact on those who share the addict's life. These could be family, loved ones, friends, work associates, and even the general public. Examples of collateral damage include the fallout of drunk driving, financial problems, and agitated or violent exchanges with the addict.

Addiction is a selfish and inconsiderate state to live in. It is centered on the gratification of the addict, with little, if any, thought to the impact addiction has on the lives of those around the addict. Addicts deftly wield defense mechanisms like denial, rationalization, and intellectualization to explain away the depth of their addiction and the damage it is doing to them and those close to them. As family and friends learn to understand these defensive strategies and refuse to work with them, the addict may go on the attack, doing whatever is necessary to maintain their ties to their addiction.

Addicts have an uncanny way of misdirecting people, shifting the conversation, and in general, keeping people from holding them accountable to anything they are doing or should be doing. Some of the defensive strategies addicts use to keep family members and friends at bay are seen in these responses:

- "I have no idea what you're talking about."

- "What I'm doing has nothing to do with you."

- "You're making too much out of this. It's not that bad."

- "I can control this anytime I want to."

- "It's my life, and I have the right to do as I choose."

- "I'm not the problem, you are."

- "Get out of my face, or I'll show you what a problem is."

All these defenses prioritize the addict's pleasure while disregarding the collateral damage.

If you are a family member, friend, or associate of an addict, and their addiction affects your life, it is essential to understand how to address both the addict and the addiction. Though you may want the addiction to stop and the addict to be more considerate of your feelings, focusing on stopping them from continuing in the addiction cannot be your primary concern. You must focus on your own physical, intellectual, emotional, and spiritual health first. You cannot help someone else unless you, yourself, are healthy enough to do so.

Addicts are master strategists. If you attempt to focus your efforts on ending the addiction, they will focus their efforts on keeping you from doing so. An addict is usually willing to go much farther in trying to maintain their addiction than you are in trying to stop them. This is why 12-step programs encourage family and friends of addicts to go to meetings, so they can learn all about addiction and about how to keep themselves healthy enough to avoid the devastation the addiction can cause.

At The Center of Things

Addicts have an uncanny way of turning the significant people in their lives into prisoners who put the addict at the center of their world and make them feel as though their sole purpose on this earth is to serve their needs. Codependency is defined as *a dysfunctional relationship dynamic where one person assumes the role of "the giver," sacrificing their own needs and well-being for the sake of the other, "the taker."* See Psychology Today https://www.psychologytoday.com/us/basics/codependency. It can leave your sense of self-worth and emotions entirely dependent on someone else.

The signs of codependency are:

- Compulsive attention to someone

- Fear of abandonment

- Lack of outside support

- Weak sense of self

- Self-doubt

- Resentment

In addition to turning you into a slave and someone with little to no self-respect and self-esteem, codependency helps keep the addiction alive. It enables the addict to continue in their abusive and self-centered way of living. Addicts need people to support their addiction and to address all the responsibilities that they, themselves, have abandoned. They tear you down, make you believe you need them, and in the process, do everything they can to make them happy while their addiction destroys them and everyone close to them. One of the most important items on your recovery checklist should be learning how to remove the addict from the center of your world and rebuild your own self-respect and self-esteem. As you will see, you are not the weak person you thought you were, and people are waiting to help you.

THE 7 STEPS TO AVOID COLLATERAL DAMAGE AND REMAIN HEALTHY

1. **NEVER PERSONALIZE THE ADDICTION**. The addiction is not about you. It's about the addict. As the addict becomes increasingly dependent on the drug or behavior, family members and friends tend to become co-addicted, putting the addict and their behaviors at the center of their world and doing their best to try to fix them. This is not your addiction; it's theirs. They are the ones who are sick, not you. Don't personalize the addiction, and don't make the addict your primary focus.

2. **NEVER MAKE AN ADDICTION A SECRET.** Keeping the addiction secret to try to protect the addict, yourself, and your family can put everyone at risk because doing so leaves you with no viable solutions, so you are destined to repeat the same addiction-controlled behaviors every day. It's important to get help. Let those you trust in. Let them know what is happening so they can support you. Contact a professional counselor if you need one. Attend a 12-step meeting for family members such as Al-Anon, Over-eaters Anonymous, etc. Talk to a clergyperson from your place of worship. Do whatever you can to enlist willing help that can see what you're experiencing with fresh eyes.

3. **TAKE STOCK OF WHAT YOU ARE DOING.** This is where you get honest with yourself. Ask yourself questions like, "What is going on in my life?" "How am I reacting?" "What things am I doing as part of this addiction?" It's also where you ask yourself, "What can I do differently?" You don't need the answers immediately; You just have to ask the questions. This is all about taking your mind off autopilot and not just blindly moving through your day. It is important to infuse your life with conscious thoughts that questions your decisions and how you are making them. These are the general questions. Then, refer back to step #2 and let others help you with the circumstances specific to what is happening in your life.

4. **CONSIDER SEEKING A HIGHER POWER.** Twelve-step programs have successfully communicated that a power greater than oneself can restore sanity. For some people, this power is God. Others choose different paths, such as the universe or the 12-step rooms. It doesn't matter what you choose, but understand that you cannot do this alone and will not be alone if you choose to get help. You can investigate the concept of a higher power online by talking to someone in a 12-step program or by attending one meeting to see what the program is all about. You have nothing to lose by taking this step.

5. **UNDERSTAND AND ACCEPT THE FACT THAT YOU ARE POWER-LESS OVER SOMEONE ELSE'S ADDICTION.** This is a hard concept

for many people to understand, especially those who are caregivers and fixers. People don't like surrendering their lives to someone else, and this applies tenfold to the addict. **YOU DO NOT HAVE THE POWER TO STOP THEIR ADDICTION,** and the sooner you understand that the faster you can turn your attention to getting the help you need to keep the addiction from taking over your life and restore the health that the addict's addiction has stolen from you.

6. **TAKE ADVANTAGE OF THE CAMARADERIE AND BE IN SERVICE OF OTHERS**. Addicts and their addictions take prisoners. You are one of those prisoners. The way to reduce the impact of the addiction in your life is to bond closely with other people who understand the addiction, who may have experienced the effects of living with or being closely associated with an addict, and who have the network and knowledge to help you restore sanity into your life. While involving yourself with these people and their programs, you will be provided the opportunity to help others. This helps you to remove some of that codependency that has plagued your life while helping you feel that you are still a viable part of humanity and that you have much to offer.

7. **MAKE THE CALL**. Again, no one comes through addiction alone. Put your pride aside and be willing to let other people help you. You can start with family and friends who are not part of the addiction problem. You can also contact a professional counselor with experience in treating families with addiction problems. Another way to address the problem is to contact the closest support group for the particular addiction you are dealing with. You will find them on the Internet along with telephone numbers for addiction help. Reach out. Bring others into your life who can help you with this problem. Never feel as though you are not worthy of the help because you are, and those who can help you are waiting for you.

Getting Support—Codependency in Check

Throughout this book, I have stressed the importance of not keeping the addiction secret and seeking and accepting help from those individuals who understand the dynamics of addiction and can support you through the movement from addiction to recovery. Collateral damage, especially for family members, can be life-altering to the point that it devastates a family. It is so important to be willing to reach out and allow others who have been through the addiction wars to share their experience with you and help you provide that road map to a healthy life without the addiction at the center of your world. The best supports for family members of addicts are AlAnon https://al-anon.org/ and Nar-Anon https://al-anon.org/. Also, by referring back to the helplines I have listed at the end of each addiction chapter, you will find the support necessary to help you through that particular addiction affecting the addict and those of you close to them. Let these people help you. The support services can be instrumental in helping you understand what codependency and enabling are and how to help you disconnect from the tendency to put the addict at the center of your world.

IN PERSPECTIVE

If you are addicted to a drug or activity, the work to become sober and stay that way can be challenging, and it never ends. However, as long as you remain consistent with your program, open and trusting of the process and the people helping you, and willing to do what it takes to achieve and maintain sobriety, that happy, healthy life you've been hoping for can be yours. Keep your life pace slow, be honest with those who are helping you and with yourself, stay away from the games that maintain the addiction, and work with your program and the people close to you on a daily basis.

The addicted person in your life may be in the throes of a horrible addiction. However, that does not mean that you have to remain a prisoner of that addiction. As with anything in life, it is a matter of perspective. You must keep the people, places, and things that enter your life from becoming personal, overly emotional, and out of perspective. Addiction has become a significant problem in your life, but that does not mean there is no way out of it.

You have no control over what the addict does. You never have, and you never will. However, you do have control over your thoughts and actions, whether it is about addiction or anything else in your life. Gaining the proper perspective about addiction sets the stage for choices that will restore health and happiness in your world while at the same time keeping you from being pulled down by the addict and their harmful choices. It is difficult to watch someone you care about destroy themselves, but it can be even more devastating to remain on the sinking ship with them.

No one says that you or anyone else needs to be involved with the addict's potentially life-destroying addiction. You can do your best to help the addict, but their willingness to accept your help is their choice. Addiction and the way addicts think and behave have a way of beating family members and loved ones down. It can make you believe that you are caught on the addiction hamster's wheel and that there is no way off of it. This is so far from the truth. Keep in mind that you do not have the addiction. Though you may be in the throes of a life-consuming addiction, you are still a good person worthy of help, and there are people with open arms waiting to help you through this. If you are a family member, a loved one, or a significant other involved with an addicted person, you are worthy of the same help. Make the call. Get the help you need!

 ## TIME TO TAKE ACTION

1. Never personalize the addiction. It is the addict's problem. Focus on yourself and what you need to do to get help.

2. Pay close attention to the "7 Steps to Avoid Collateral Damage and Remain Healthy." They are an introduction to help you begin to make the changes you need to survive the addict's addiction.

3. Identify people you think can help you. They may be support people, family, friends, clergy, and professional counselors. Make the call to at least one of them to get things started.

4. A 12-step program can be a lifesaver not only for addicts but for their families. Keep things in perspective. It is much easier to attend a 12-step meeting than it is to continue to be part of a life-destroying addiction. Try to get past yourself on this one. Attend the meeting.

5. Think about working with the concept of a higher power. If you are unsure what to do with this part of the program, talk to others using one. Your higher power will be far more potent than the addict's addiction.

6. Be willing to reach out to a support group to help you understand the addiction and what you need to do to keep it from taking over your world.

7. Remember that you are worth all the time and effort it takes to help you through whatever the addict's addiction has cost in your life. Never look at yourself as anything but worthy, and let people in.

 ## DRIVING IT HOME

Addiction often destroys the lives of the addict and those close to them, but this needn't be the case for you. Understand that while an addiction destroys the addict emotionally and intellectually, it has the same impact on those close to them. Caught in the addictive dilemma, family members can feel broken, have difficulty making decisions, and can quickly get caught in the negative swell the addiction causes. The addict is the person with the addiction, and they must be willing to accept help to make the changes they need to live a happy and healthy life. You are not less worthy because they have a problem. Getting help can restore your sanity, and it just may be the first step in helping the person with the addiction since you will no longer be feeding into the addiction end, enabling the addict's dysfunctional decisions and behaviors. Be willing to get the help you need. You can do this!

YOUR DECLARATION IS: *I will not do this alone. I will let others in, and I will get the help I need to be healthy!*

 ## ONWARD

In the next chapter, I will explore the first step of recovery. I will look at a decision that must be "etched in stone." I will talk about the pull back into the addiction and what is necessary to be strong enough to resist it.

CHAPTER 24

◇◇◇◇◇◇◇◇◇◇◇◇◇

The Decision—
Getting Down and Dirty

There is no "almost" and no second-guessing. The decision to live
is an either-or enterprise. You decide to live or not.

PROCESSES TO EMPLOY: Brutal Honesty, I Over E, Present-
Understand-Fix, Slowing Down Life's Pace, Internal Focus, Fact-
Finding, Honesty, Patience, Truth-Telling, Belief, Listening, Trust,
Intelligent Decision-Making, Life Inventory, Conflict Resolution,
Reduction of Destination Living, Goal-Setting, Living in the
Moment, One-Day-at-a-Time-Living, Boundary-Setting, Warm
Communication, Settling Past Issues, Risk-Taking, Be Comfortable
with Being Uncomfortable

ACCOUNTABILITY CAN BE THE BITTER PILL in an otherwise do-what-
you-want world. It's one thing to say you will do something, but holding
yourself accountable and making it happen is another. It's even more
difficult to hold yourself accountable consistently. Each day surrounds us
with decisions to make, followed by the accountability demanded to turn
the decision into action. We often avoid making healthy decisions since
we know what must follow is for us to be accountable for those decisions,
and accountability demands action.

Making the right decisions to address an addiction, whether you are
the addict or the addict's family member, requires action to turn that
decision into reality. The action demands that you be accountable for the

steps you take to execute your decision. You know there is a problem, and something must be done about it. You also know there can be resistance to your decision or, at the very least, discomfort associated with making the change.

In the less critical situations in our lives, not being accountable doesn't have quite the blowback as in more serious life circumstances. Addiction is one of those serious life circumstances. In recovery, there is no halfway, no leeway, and no wiggle room. Addiction can have a devastating impact on the addict, and it can be just as devastating for family members. If you are going to address addiction, whether you are the addict or the family member, it demands a cut-and-dry decision. You decide to become a sober person if you are the addict, or if you are a family member or someone close to the addict, you decide that you will no longer allow the collateral damage from the addict to touch your life. Cut-and-dry decisions like these demand a level of accountability that is blunt and straight to the point.

DECISIONS, DECISIONS

Deciding to remove oneself from the addiction merry-go-round can be a difficult and multifaceted undertaking. Deciding to leave the addiction and get healthy is only the first decision. Many will follow. The most important are:

FOR THE ADDICT: The first decision is to stop indulging in the drug or activity of choice.

FOR FAMILY MEMBERS AND LOVED ONES: The first decision is whether to stay in the relationship with the addict.

FOR THE ADDICT: Understanding that you are powerless over the addiction, your second decision is to begin your one-day-at-a-time program to avoid the substance or activity.

FOR FAMILY MEMBERS AND LOVED ONES: Your second decision is to understand that you are powerless over the addiction and that you cannot change the addict. That person must make that decision for themselves.

FOR THE ADDICT: Third, you must decide who is going to be involved in the process of helping you remove the addictive substance or activity from your life.

FOR FAMILY MEMBERS AND LOVED ONES: Your third decision is whose advice to seek in understanding the addictive process and getting started in the first step of your recovery from the addict's influence.

FOR THE ADDICT: Your fourth decision is whether you are going to follow the advice of those who will help you stop your addiction or if you are going to choose to do things your way.

FOR FAMILY MEMBERS: Your fourth decision is whether you are willing to follow the advice of those helping you, even though you may feel uncomfortable and put into a position to make choices that could drastically alter the condition of your life and those close to you and the life of the addict as it relates to you.

FOR THE ADDICT: Your fifth decision is to either go to counseling or an inpatient program, if necessary and to include that 12-step program or other support programs in your life.

FOR FAMILY MEMBERS AND LOVED ONES: Your fifth decision, even though it is the addict's addiction that caused the problems, is whether support groups and 12-step programs are something you are willing to undertake for yourself.

FOR THE ADDICT: Your sixth decision is whether to let others know that you are an addict and that you are trying to avoid the drug or activity that has consumed your life.

FOR FAMILY MEMBERS AND LOVED ONES: Your sixth decision is whether to tell others close to you that there is addiction in your family and that there may be some new boundaries or procedures you must follow to remain healthy.

FOR THE ADDICT: Your seventh decision is to be honest about the damage you have done to family, friends, loved ones, and significant others.

FOR FAMILY MEMBERS AND LOVED ONES: Your seventh decision is holding the addict accountable enough to be honest and make amends to you and anyone else who has been hurt. This is essential so that neither you nor the addict repeat dysfunctional behaviors.

FOR THE ADDICT: Your eighth decision will be the willingness to put yourself at the mercy of others, such as counselors and 12-step program members, who can guide you through the initial stages of recovery and help you maintain the program necessary to live a healthy, sober life.

FOR FAMILY MEMBERS AND LOVED ONES: Your eighth decision is to continue to learn about addiction, yourself, and possibly your codependency, and to listen to those who can help take you through the steps necessary to maintain your recovery, such as counselors and 12-step program members.

FOR THE ADDICT: Your ninth decision is whether you're willing to make your recovery a lifetime program that you will invest yourself in and never stop.

FOR FAMILY MEMBERS AND LOVED ONES: Your ninth decision is whether to make your recovery program a lifetime investment that will never stop.

FOR THE ADDICT: Your tenth decision is to recognize that life is dynamic and will continue to change and that you must continue to grow in your recovery program and stay close to your support people.

FOR FAMILY MEMBERS AND LOVED ONES: Your tenth decision is whether to accept that even though both you and the addict may be in recovery, your life will continue to change, and your continued involvement in your support program is essential to maintain your recovery and the gains you have made.

Following through on these decisions is crucial if you are going to put active addiction in the rearview mirror. There is no destination you will arrive at where the addiction will be completely in the past and where you will not need to continue to address it with support and counseling. Those who understand this have a much easier time making these ten decisions. If you never choose to enter a recovery program, the addiction will be a lifetime enterprise. Likewise, if you plan to lead a healthy life free of active addiction, your recovery program is also a lifetime endeavor.

GETTING UNCOMFORTABLE TO BE COMFORTABLE

If anyone tells you that the initial decision to stop using (if you are the addict) or to make any of the decisions an addict's family members must make is going to be easy, you are being misled. Nothing about addiction is ever easy. That includes:

➤ The decision to get help to stop using can include detoxification services, inpatient programming, counseling, and support services (for the addict).

➤ The decision to remove oneself from the addiction may also include counseling and support programming (for family members, loved ones, and significant others).

➤ The decision to continually refrain from actively pursuing the drug or activity of choice (for the addict).

➤ The decision to set boundaries, to no longer allow the addict to make empty promises, and to begin the process of setting boundaries and making good decisions (for family members, loved ones, and significant others).

➤ The decision to embrace a lifestyle that does not include the drug or activity of choice as well as any replacement addictions, to live without it, and to build a life that will continue to include counseling and/or support services (for the addict).

➤ The decision to use a tougher form of love, to no longer make the addict the center of one's life, and to continue pursuing counseling and support services that can help maintain a healthy lifestyle (for family, loved ones, and significant others).

In the initial stages of recovery, even the best-laid plans can fall by the wayside, so making all the decisions and the changes inherent in executing those decisions is uncomfortable and often painful. Going into recovery requires that the addict, their family, and those close to them understand that although there may be light at the end of the tunnel, there is much work to do and much to fix, and the recovery process can, at times, be difficult.

This is why having a network behind you in the early stages of recovery is so important. These people have often been through the addiction wars and understand what you will be facing. They can help you avoid the pitfalls and slips often inherent in recovery. They understand that you are going to get uncomfortable, that you'll experience pain on a variety of levels, and that you will be afraid. Once again, nothing about addiction is easy, but nothing about addiction is impossible. You will experience a period of discomfort, but as long as you stay accountable and stick with the program, good things can happen.

Look at it this way: If you're a cigarette smoker and you have smoked a pack of cigarettes every day for twenty years, you might experience acute anxiety, headaches, and severe cravings without nicotine, especially during the first week or two. After that, your mind may still want a cigarette, but the discomfort that comes with the physical withdrawal is markedly reduced. This is the way all addictions work. The initial stages of recovery are difficult, and there is a withdrawal not only from the drug but also from the lifestyle that accompanies it.

The important decision is to leave the addiction, followed by the decision to let others help you. Many people have survived addiction and have gone on to lead happy and fulfilled lives. You can, too. The key is to decide to stop what you are doing, get help and listen to those helping you, follow through with their direction, and make your recovery program the cornerstone for your new life.

FOLLOWING THROUGH

Everyone makes decisions every day. Good decisions are made by acquiring the necessary information about the problem, prioritizing that information, and devising a plan to solve the problem based on the information gathered. All too often, loved ones do not take the time to educate themselves enough to address the problem caused by the addict's addiction. Addicts caught in the clutches of the addiction rarely have the ability to gather the information they need about the addiction.

Once you have decided to stop letting the addiction affect your life, whether you are the addict or the family member, loved one, or significant other, you must follow through and stay consistent with the program that is outlined for you. Suppose you are moving to a foreign land and do not speak the language very well. In that case, you might hire a guide to show you how to navigate the new territory, keep you away from places that could be problematic, explain things to you when you become confused, and be there for you for all your needs until you understand how to take care of yourself. This is the way addiction works. Your guides are your counselors, 12-step members, medical professionals, and others who have extensive experience with addiction and primarily with recovery. They will teach you how to navigate your new recovery territory, keep you away from the potential pitfalls that could lead you back to addiction or codependent issues, and explain all the various parts of the program to help make your recovery easier and more efficient. They will be there for you until you understand how to navigate your new world.

This is why nothing about addiction is easy, but everything about recovery has a solution. Following through means acknowledging that you will not do this alone and being comfortable with that. It means making decisions and holding yourself accountable for doing what those decisions demand. It means getting uncomfortable but sticking with it and pushing through those difficult times with the help of people who love you and are willing to support you. It means following through and staying consistent in your recovery program for the rest of your life. Those willing to do this will find that life can take on an entirely new meaning, and you will find your happiness there.

Time to Take Action

1. If you are an addict, decide to stop using your drug or activity of choice.

2. Understand that the decision and the willingness to get help from a professional addictions counselor and a support program can help you define and establish your new recovery territory. Involve yourself with someone who can help you start the process of recovery.

3. Follow the decisions listed earlier in this chapter to the best of your ability. They will help you to begin the recovery program you need to leave the addiction behind.

4. Remember that you are entering a recovery program. It's not a cure; recovery is a lifetime enterprise. Those who continue to work their program drastically increase their chances of success and their potential to be happy.

5. Decide to leave the addiction for good. There is no halfway in recovery. You either have it or you don't. Make the decision, get the help, follow through, and never quit.

 ## Driving It Home

Two kinds of people enter recovery programs: Some steadfastly embrace all the components of recovery, regardless of how much effort they need to put into the program. Others have a difficult time following through, either because they are still drawn to the addiction or because they are unwilling to do the work the recovery process demands. If you truly want to be happy and free of the active phase of the addiction, be willing to do the work and embrace everything that goes along with acquiring and maintaining your sobriety. You will connect with parts of yourself and the world around you that were previously unavailable to you. As you do, you will define the gift that is your new life.

YOUR DECLARATION IS: *I will make the necessary decisions, listen to people who know how to help me, and follow through with my recovery program for the rest of my life!*

 ONWARD

In the next chapter, I will examine how arrogance hinders a healthy recovery process and how humility is necessary to survive one's addiction. I will also explore the willingness to accept help from those who have been where you are.

CHAPTER 25

◇◇◇◇◇◇◇◇◇◇◇◇◇

Getting Help—
Letting Them In

*It is where arrogance and humility trade places, and the willingness
to embrace the wisdom of those who know the way is born.*

PROCESSES TO EMPLOY: Brutal Honesty, I Over E, Present-
Understand-Fix, Slowing Down Life's Pace, Internal Focus,
Fact-Finding, Honesty, Patience, Truth-Telling, Belief, Listening,
Trust, Reduction of Destination Living, Goal-Setting, Living in
the Moment, One-Day-at-a-Time Living, Boundary-Setting,
Warm Communication, Settling Past Issues, Risk-Taking,
Be Comfortable with Being Uncomfortable, Humility

ADDICTION IS ALL TOO OFTEN A SECRETIVE WAY OF LIFE. Addicts
are very slow to admit that there could be a problem with their chosen
substance or activity. Family members are often embarrassed and afraid
of what might happen if they disclose what is occurring and can become
addiction coconspirators. They hide what the addict is doing and also
what it is doing to them. This creates fertile ground for the addiction to
grow and makes it difficult for others who are willing to help.

It is so important to let others in to help, as I have stressed in the
previous chapter. It is difficult to make decisions that are in the best
interest of both the addict and family members when everyone is con-
tinuously caught in the downward spiral and hiding what is happening.
Addiction can change everything about the way a family operates. Relationships suffer, there is often significant financial loss, communication

is typically avoided, and in some cases, abuse and physical harm are a distinct possibility.

It feels embarrassing to let others know what is happening because then they will also know that you've long been wearing a mask to hide the fact that yours is a family where an addict lives and that things are far from perfect. We all like others to believe that we are happy and doing well. We fear becoming the focal point of gossip, and we fear that others will look down on us. No one likes to be thought of as that family down the street with the dirty little secret. Though this may not be what will happen, it is very easy for our minds to create that scenario.

OUT OF THE CLOSET

At least in the short run, secrets keep others from knowing who we are and what is happening in our lives. If we are successful secret keepers, we avoid the embarrassment of having others know that our families have severe problems. It keeps us from feeling vulnerable to unsympathetic and merciless people. It allows us to navigate a world that can be cruel and unforgiving without surrendering the more intimate details of our lives. It protects us and reduces the potential impact of vicious attacks from other people.

The unfortunate side effect of keeping secrets is that we remain prisoners behind the masks we create. We must be constantly on guard and ready to fend off potential assaults, and we live in a state of emotional paranoia, doing everything we can to keep others from understanding who we are and what we are experiencing. Leaving the addiction closet is an admission that we don't measure up to our perception of how happy and put together other people are. Hiding an addiction is hiding who we are, whether we are the addict or the family member of the addict. Whichever you are, no one wants this secret to become common knowledge.

However, if you are going to get help to stop the damage the addiction is doing, you have to come out of the addiction closet and stop protecting the secret that nurtures this horrible way of living. As I mentioned previously, there will be an uncomfortable period in the early stages of recovery. People are going to learn that you are either addicted or are living with an addict. That may not feel good initially, but the goal is to stop the addiction and get healthy. What others say or think does not matter. Would you rather protect your secret and continue to live a life of pain at the hands of the addiction, or are you willing to step out from the shadows, get the help you need, and begin to live a happy and healthy life?

You needn't broadcast the fact that you are either addicted or that you are living with an addict. You won't tell the world every horrible little detail about what you have been living with. You are simply going to ask other people for help, which, by definition, breaks the veil of secrecy and puts you in a position to move past the addiction. Others may find out that you are doing this, but the truth of the matter is that addiction is hard to keep under wraps forever. Sooner or later, they will find out something. It makes far more sense to have them find out that you were living with an addiction, that you had the courage to take the necessary steps to understand the problem, and that you got the help you needed to address it. Once again, it is not about what anyone else thinks or says. It is about you getting help for a severe and life-threatening problem.

TAKING THE FIRST STEPS

The hardest part of addressing any problem is to know what to do first and how to do it. As I mentioned in Chapter 24, you start addressing the addiction by deciding to get help. Nothing happens until you make that decision. Once you do, there is no turning back. You must decide that this is what you will do, that nothing can stop you, and that you won't second-guess yourself or find reasons to put off the decision or negotiate your way into a process that keeps you comfortable and not fully committed to recovery.

Having decided to get help for the addiction, here are the steps you need to take to start your recovery process:

1. Make an appointment with your primary care physician to determine if any physical concerns must be addressed.

2. Decide whom you will ask for help and make an initial appointment with that person or attend your first support meeting.

3. Present as much information as possible to those who will help you.

4. Be willing to attend your second counseling session or support meeting.

5. Be open to taking the advice of the people you are asking to help you.

I will expand on each of these steps to help you more clearly understand the process involved. Initially, since this is unknown territory for you, taking your first steps can be difficult. It can be an emotional time for you, so it's a little easier if you understand exactly how to proceed as you take your first steps.

1. **MAKE AN APPOINTMENT WITH YOUR PRIMARY CARE PHYSICIAN TO DETERMINE IF ANY PHYSICAL CONCERNS NEED TO BE ADDRESSED.** Determining who to call to start your recovery program can be intimidating, so start with your primary care physician. Make an appointment with your doctor and give them as much information as possible about what is happening. This should include the type of addiction you are dealing with, how long it has been happening, any physical problems that have developed, and your family history, particularly as it relates to addiction. Your primary care physician will ask questions related to the addiction and will usually have a list of addiction specialists, rehabilitation centers, support programs, and other professionals available to help you start the process. At times, obtaining an appointment with your doctor may take a while. As you are waiting, be willing to call one of the hotline numbers to gather the information you need to get your program started.

2. **DECIDE WHOM YOU WILL ASK FOR HELP.** If your primary care physician gives you an initial contact person, call that person. That person might be a professional counselor, a 12-step program contact, or another professional with an addiction background. Make an appointment for an initial consultation or be willing to attend one support meeting on a trial basis. Taking this step helps you in two ways: 1) It helps you make the first step to take the problem out of the family and into the hands of a professional or support person, and 2) It gives you a direction that includes other people to help you and more

of the relevant information you need to understand the addiction and how to move past it.

3. **PRESENT AS MUCH INFORMATION AS POSSIBLE TO THOSE WHO WILL SUPPORT YOU.** This will help them formulate a program that meets your specific needs. Anyone's ability to help you depends on how much accurate information you give them. You don't need to have all the answers, but you have to be willing to answer questions honestly and provide facts so they may understand what you have been living with and help you take the initial steps to begin the recovery process.

4. **BE WILLING TO ATTEND EITHER YOUR SECOND COUNSELING SESSION OR YOUR SECOND SUPPORT MEETING.** Even though you have taken the right steps to connect with people who will help you in the initial stages of the recovery program, once you are there, it will still be new territory, and it can be somewhat intimidating. It is very easy to turn away at this point and try to convince yourself that you didn't get much out of it, to say it's not for you, or to make some other excuse not to go. Remember, even moving in the right direction, including a program that can save your life and help make it a happy place to live, can be uncomfortable. It is stepping out of what you considered a comfort zone and into an unknown way to live with new people you don't know yet. Tell them if you are having a difficult time, and let them gently guide you as you progress in the program.

5. **BE OPEN TO TAKING THE ADVICE OF THE PEOPLE YOU ARE ASKING TO HELP YOU.** Getting help for addiction carries all the classic approach-avoidance feelings. The advice is to slow down and keep your emotions from overriding your logical brain. Be willing to trust these people enough to get to know them and to understand what they are telling you to do. No one is expecting you to understand the information immediately. There are no tests to determine if you do. You are attempting to step out of an addictive way of life and into a recovery program that can have tremendous positive effects on your life. Try to relax as much as possible, confide in these people, and let them guide you through the program.

ROOM TO BREATHE

Living with an addiction can be a stifling experience; sometimes, it's difficult to catch your breath. In its mildest cases, addiction comes with a loss of finances, verbal arguments, compromised family time, and priorities being left unaddressed. In the more serious cases, it could lead to loss of homes, loss of health, severe cases of abuse, and death. Addiction does not discriminate; it has no boundaries, and it respects no one. Addicts are often caught in the obsession that drives them to the addiction. It can destroy their lives and have a serious impact on those close to them. Family members never know exactly what to expect, are always prepared for the worst, and are often exhausted by the emotional tug-of-war that defines their lives. Just having a moment to catch one's breath is a godsend.

Addicts and family members alike pray for an end to this vicious cycle and say they are willing to do anything to make it stop. However, when the time comes to follow through and pursue a course of recovery that includes people to help them through the process, they can struggle. For those who are willing to stretch beyond the clutches of the addiction and reach out to others who have experience or expertise in addiction to guide them into the beginnings of a recovery process, there is hope. They can finally catch their breath, knowing that they don't have to do this alone and that others are there whenever they need help.

As you will see in the next chapter, asking for help can be difficult for two reasons:

➤ It demands that you surrender control part of your life to someone you do not yet know.

➤ It demands that you *trust someone* who knows how to help you but with whom you do not yet have a history.

Keep this in mind. As you take these initial steps into the recovery process, you begin removing yourself from a life that is often suffocating, abusive, and unrelenting. You are making this decision because you understand that if you continue to stay in the clutches of the addiction, you will remain unhappy, abused, and emotionally exhausted.

Allowing other people to help you can set the stage for a life that can be significantly more productive, happier, and more peaceful. To make this happen, however, you need to take the initial steps to gain a better understanding of addiction and the treatment alternatives that are available to you.

So, those decisions I discussed in Chapter 24 and the willingness to let others help you are the combination you need to begin your recovery. Knowing that they must do something to stop the damage the addiction is doing and to take control of their lives, many people never decide to get help. The decisions are the necessary first steps, but the follow-through is equally important. Decide to do what it takes to restore order and sanity to your life. Be willing to let others in and accept the advice and assistance they are willing to provide. If you do, your journey into a life of recovery from addiction can finally begin.

As I have reiterated throughout this book, nothing about addiction is easy, and no one says recovery will be. However, by choosing to get help, you will be dedicating yourself to a program with a solid and positive forward progression. People with the experience and expertise to help you open new doors that can lead to happiness are waiting for you. Make the decisions, follow through, and begin what can become the best part of your life.

⏱ TIME TO TAKE ACTION

1. Decide to open up about your addiction problem. Be willing to let others in to help you.

2. Follow the steps to start your recovery process, as listed earlier in this chapter.

3. After you identify the people who will help you, schedule your first meeting with them to help you understand what you need to do and to help them understand how they can help you.

4. Listen to what the people who are helping you say. Follow their advice and continue to attend their meetings.

DRIVING IT HOME

Your decision to "come out of the closet" about your addiction problem may be the most difficult decision you may ever make, but it is also the most important decision you may ever make. No important decisions are ever easy, and the following work will be involved and span the rest of your life. However, involving yourself in a recovery program is so much better than being stuck in the addiction's clutches. This is your real decision: "Am I willing to start the recovery process and stay committed for the rest of my life, or am I willing to stay in the clutches of the addiction for the rest of my life?" Everything you do hereafter will follow that decision. Choose recovery. You can do this!

YOUR DECLARATION IS: *I will let others in, listen to them, and accept the commitment to a lifetime recovery program!*

 ## ONWARD

In the next chapter, I will discuss surrendering to a program that can rescue you from your addiction and help restore your life to health and sanity. I will look at 12-step programs as an addition to a counseling program.

◇◇◇◇◇◇◇◇◇◇◇◇

CHAPTER 26

Taking the Steps— Powerful Surrender

It is where powerlessness, surrender, and the understanding of a power greater than yourself wrap themselves around you, changing your life forever.

PROCESSES TO EMPLOY: Brutal Honesty, I Over E, Present-Understand-Fix, Slowing Down Life's Pace, Internal Focus, Fact-Finding, Honesty, Patience, Truth-Telling, Belief, Listening, Trust, Reduction of Destination Living, Goal-Setting, Living in the Moment, One-Day-at-a-Time Living, Boundary-Setting, Warm Communication, Settling Past Issues, Risk-Taking, Be Comfortable with Being Uncomfortable, Humility, Surrender

---

THE TRADITIONAL DEFINITION OF "SURRENDER" IS *to give over to the power, control, or possession of another, especially by force.* Unfortunately, this is exactly how we tend to view surrender in the context of addiction recovery. Many of us have read about surrender in novels, been taught about it in history classes, heard of military operations forcing the enemy to surrender, and seen it often in the movies we watch. The common theme is that surrender means *unwillingly* giving up control to varying degrees to some opposing force.

I will offer a very different definition of "surrender." This is the one you will use in your recovery program, and it will be essential to start the program and to keep it working for you for the rest of your life.

*Surrender is letting go of people, places, and things that weigh us down, stag-
nate us, may cause fear and pain, and hold us back from the necessary changes
in our lives.* It opens the door to more powerful forces that can restore
our lives to peace and sanity and connect us with our higher power. The
connection with our higher power paves the way for potentially limitless
thought and action and introduces us to the serenity that is crucial for
healthy living.

CONCEDING TO A FORCE
GREATER THAN OURSELVES

Humans are a species still connected to primal drives. Living has always
been survival of the fittest, and surrender does not seem to have a place
in that design. It is generally important for people to be perceived by
others as powerful because being seen as weak or powerless can leave one
feeling vulnerable. So, due to these primal drives, it is assumed that the
way to "survive" is to be powerful, to let others know you are powerful,
and to never back down or surrender.

Surrender has always had a converse relationship with survival. If
we include surrender in our life plan, we assume that others will perceive
us as weak. This archaic mentality keeps us connected to primal ways of
thinking and behaving and stands in the way of the evolution to higher-order thinking and behaving.

Surrender in the traditional framework demands the loss of will
and control and, in the end, severely compromises freedom of thought.
It assumes that the force we surrender to may usurp all we are and
everything we have since that traditional definition calls for giving our
power, control, and possessions to another, stronger entity. The traditional definition can apply in situations that call for survival, such as
military skirmishes and battles, conditions related to potential physical
harm, and attempts to be controlled by others. However, surrender,
as it applies to recovery, demands an entirely different perspective. In
recovery, it is essential to let go of those people, places, and things that
weigh us down and connect us to the obsessive-compulsive nature of
addiction.

Addiction, by its very nature, does not let go of anything that may interfere with the continued use of the drug or activity of choice. Though addicts are quite adept at discarding people and responsibilities from their lives in favor of their addiction, they do not discard anything that can protect the addiction and keep others from threatening their relationship with it. When you look closely at the definition of "surrender" I presented, you will notice that addiction causes addicts to remain close to people and things and in places that weigh them down, stagnate them and hold them back from the changes that are so necessary for their lives. At the same time, the addiction instigates a disconnection from their higher power and that limitless thought and behavior that is so deeply connected to it.

SURRENDERING TO THE POWER

The traditional design for surrender assumes that we will acquiesce to a power that supersedes our own, will take what we have, and is wrought with negative energy, coercion, and pain. It has no connection to a higher power with positive energy and no potential for growth, higher-order thought, peace, or serenity. It is surrender by force and is to be avoided at all costs. Avoiding this kind of surrender is understandable; one is giving up not only possessions but, in many cases, their freedom. As I define it, "surrender" has nothing to do with negative energy, coercion, and pain. It is letting go of what can cause harm to the addicts and those close to them and embracing a power source that is positive, loving, and peaceful. It is the letting go of what is negative to embrace what is positive.

We often struggle with letting go of one part of our life to embrace a new chapter because we don't know what that new chapter will look like. It is an unfamiliar territory, one that we have yet to travel. We struggle toward something we cannot see and touch. It is difficult enough to leave what is familiar and invest our intellects and our emotions in something new, but when that new territory is undefined, we can feel lost and without direction. This is one of the reasons family members stay in relationships with addicts. Though the new territory may include the potential for growth and happiness, it demands that we leave what we know and pursue something unknown, undefined, and often overwhelming.

THE TRUST FACTOR

Embarking into new territory without a guide can make that new venture seem like an obstacle course with all kinds of hidden dangers. Even though the addiction prison could be a painful place to live, you know the terrain, and you know how to deal with every little twist and turn it offers. It is painful, but you understand that pain. You know what to expect and where you fit into the addiction scenario. Taking your first steps into recovery requires a leap of faith, and it most certainly requires trust. You must trust yourself, believe that you are making the right decision, and trust those you enlist to assist you on your journey.

Often, the people we select to help us are people we hardly know. We choose them because they have experience or expertise in recovery from addiction, and we need them to guide us into this uncharted territory. However, how often do we trust the people we do not know with our lives? How often do we tell strangers our most intimate details, trusting that they will keep those details in confidence and use them to guide us away from the addiction and into a new and healthy way of living?

Without a doubt, recovery has much to do with trust. For many people, this is the first stumbling block following the decision to attempt to leave the addiction. These people we are trying to trust are telling us the things we don't want to hear and providing us with direction into places we are unsure we want to go. Picture this: You are caught in the proverbial dark alley. In front of you are two menacing creatures who you are sure will either hurt or kill you. Behind you is someone you do not know saying, "Come with me, and I will get you to safety." In that moment, you can either continue to move forward, which is akin to staying in the addiction, or you can trust the voice you do not know, which is promising safety.

Trust is demanded when you surrender to a higher power, to those who are helping you, and to the program they have used and are now sharing with you. This is not blind surrender. It is surrendering to life with a new plan surrounded by people who will love and guide you carefully, backed by a program with over a century of success, all under the umbrella of a higher power.

THE 7 STEPS TO POWERFUL SURRENDER

These apply to the addict and family members.

1. Understand that the decisions you have been making have not worked for you, be willing to allow others to help you, and accept that you are powerless over the addiction and what it has done to you and your life.

2. Be willing to relinquish the control you think you have over your life and allow others to help direct its course.

3. Follow the advice of the people helping you without attempting to negotiate or alter parts of that advice.

4. Be completely honest with the people who are helping you.

5. Communicate openly. There are times when your recovery program will become difficult for you, or you feel as though you want to quit. Open up about your feelings to those who are trying to help you.

6. Ask questions only when you need clarification. Do not enter into debates with people who know more than you do about what is happening to you, how to get through it, and how to reach a happy life.

7. Attend all counseling sessions and meetings in person if you can. These sessions and meetings are your lifeline to the sober and happy life waiting for you. Embrace what you hear in these meetings and counseling sessions, and do your best to follow the advice you are given.

There is no power to be found by remaining in the addiction. This is truly an oxymoron. There is no power in isolating yourself and convincing yourself that you can handle this alone. You do not have the power to protect others if you remain in the grasp of the addiction. Your ability to solve your addiction-related problems is minuscule. If that were not the case, you would have done so already.

Be willing to get help for your addiction. Don't minimize its effect on your life and those close to you. Understand the power the addiction has over you, the damage it has done to all involved, and that a program of recovery is available to you, along with the people who will always be there for you. However, this demands that you surrender to that program, to those people, and, if you can, to a power higher than yourself. In the end, you are surrendering to connect with true power. *The 12 Steps and Traditions*, by Bill W., presents the essential format that is necessary to understand and apply in most 12-step programs. You can find it at https://aa.org.au/members/three-legacies/twelve-steps/

Most 12-step programs use these steps or a variation of them. They form a rational plan to help you live a sober, healthy, productive, and loving life. One does not need to be an addict or the family member of an addict to practice the 12 steps. They are not only a program for sobriety and family health; they are a program to help anyone navigate through their lives. However, any good program is only as good as the amount of time and effort you are willing to put into it. The addiction has controlled many aspects of your life. You surrendered to the power of the addiction. Addiction takes you to the brink of disaster, and you will have dedicated a tremendous amount of time, effort, and resources to maintain this life-stealing nemesis. You must ask yourself, "Am I willing to put in the same amount of time, effort, and resources to save my life and my relationship with those close to me?"

If you can answer yes, a recovery program and helpful people are waiting to help you through this. No one can serve two masters. You will either put all your time and effort into your program, or you will remain in the clutches of the addiction, along with all the collateral damage it causes. As I have reiterated many times through this book, nothing about addiction is easy. In the early stages, your recovery can be difficult. However, if you are willing to surrender this mirage of power you thought you had to the program and the people waiting for you and, if possible, to a power higher than yourself, that peaceful life can be yours. It may be difficult, but many have done it, and so can you. You can do this. Make the call to your primary care physician or to any of the numbers listed throughout this book.

TIME TO TAKE ACTION

1. Understand the difference between the traditional definition of "surrender" and the definition I provided about surrendering to connect with true power.

2. Make the call to either an addiction counselor or the call number for a 12-step program. Attend your first session.

3. Be willing to admit that you are powerless over the addiction and that there are people and programs available who understand what you are dealing with and who are helping you through it.

4. Be willing to surrender control to those people and the recovery program they are introducing you to.

5. Don't challenge them, and be willing to listen to and take their advice.

6. Understand that this is a program for life, and be willing to make the day-to-day commitment to continue working with your recovery people and your recovery program.

 ## DRIVING IT HOME

Arrogance has a funny way of expressing itself. As opposed to an in-your-face, hostile attack, sometimes it's more subtle, unmoving, and unwilling to surrender. Sometimes, surrender is exactly what we need. We are all connected, and what one of us does can drastically affect those close to us. When life isn't working for us, it makes sense to seek out others with more wisdom and the willingness to be there for us. When fighting the addiction demon, surrender does not mean a loss of control or power—quite the opposite. You are not surrendering so someone can take all that you have. You surrender to connect with a power higher than yourself who can provide you with everything you need. Be willing to surrender the addiction to those who are helping you and to a power greater than yourself. In the end, you will understand what true power is.

YOUR DECLARATION IS: *I will surrender to the higher power and the program that can help me restore my life to peace and sanity!*

 ## ONWARD

In the next chapter, I will expand on how arrogance hinders a healthy recovery process and how humbling oneself opens the door to the help necessary to survive addiction. I will also discuss humility and gratitude, which make room for the wisdom that is essential to healthy living.

CHAPTER 27

In Recovery—The Simple Road to Wisdom

It is where the serenity to accept the things you cannot change, the courage to change the things you can, and the wisdom to know the difference become your life's guiding light.

PROCESSES TO EMPLOY: Brutal Honesty, I Over E, Present-Understand-Fix, Slowing Down Life's Pace, Internal Focus, Fact-Finding, Honesty, Patience, Truth-Telling, Belief, Listening, Trust, Reduction of Destination Living, Goal-Setting, Living in the Moment, One-Day-at-a-Time Living, Boundary-Setting, Warm Communication, Settling Past Issues, Risk-Taking, Be Comfortable with Being Uncomfortable, Humility, Gratitude

WE ARE ALL BORN WITH FREE WILL. This allows us to collect information we believe is important and make decisions based on that information. When the information-gathering process is efficient and factual, our emotions do not override our intellectual capabilities, and we have no ulterior motives. Free will can lead to decisions that can positively impact our lives. However, when life circumstances like addiction interfere with our information-gathering process, the facts can become distorted, and our free will can guide us in directions that can range from mildly disturbing to life-threatening.

Addiction is loaded with personal agendas, manipulation, lies, coercion, and meaningless displays of power. It is an example of arrogance at peak performance. I define "arrogance" as *overbearing pride and haughtiness, demonstrating a perceived position of superiority.* Those caught in the grasp of the addiction are often condescending and angry, and they firmly believe their way is the right way. They rarely listen to the positions asserted by other people and can quickly take issue with any opinion that runs contrary to their own. Arrogance is often one of the primary conditions that fuels the addiction. It's hard to accept any alternate ways of doing things when they run counter to one's own ways and threaten the continuation of the addiction.

It is almost impossible to accept the things you cannot change, have the courage to change the things you can, and know the difference between them when free will turns to arrogance. That way of thinking does not allow for the infusion of new information. Life is a dynamic endeavor; it constantly changes, and the information necessary to navigate it must be reevaluated and changed when necessary. Arrogance does not allow this process to unfold.

In Chapter 26, I discussed how important it is to be willing to listen to the people who are guiding you into your recovery, to take their advice, and to follow through with that advice. This cannot happen if arrogance is running your life. Understanding what other people are teaching us requires being humble enough to admit that we do not have all the answers, that our way is not always correct, and that what we have been doing may have caused problems for us and those close to us. Arrogance causes us to believe we have acquired enough wisdom and arrived at a station in life where no further information is necessary because we have all the answers. This is something I refer to as *naive wisdom.*

Authentic wisdom, on the other hand, is the product of our willingness to acquiesce to others and to continue to gain information that we may use to improve our lives. This wisdom helps us understand that the expertise and experience of others are necessary for us to improve our lives and that we must be humble enough to accept this information and apply it.

We often see naive arrogance with addicts. To protect the addiction, they present themselves as having all the answers, are condescending to those who challenge them, and firmly believe that they are right. As a result, they have a difficult time accepting advice that runs counter to their own. Recovering from addiction demands the willingness to accept help from others. That requires being humble enough to admit you are wrong and being willing to accept the viewpoints of others who have more experience in recovery than you do.

For family members of the addict, the arrogance is a bit more subtle, but it can also interfere with the willingness to accept help from others. This happens when family members attempt to protect the addict and what is happening at home from perceived public ridicule. It also happens when family members believe that others will not understand what is happening and that, in some fashion, they are going to help the addict recover from the addiction on their own. Though the arrogance presents differently for the addict and family members, the combination provides a strong defense to keep others out and, as a result, the addiction flourishes.

In *The Fix Yourself Handbook*, I included a chapter called "Wisdom and the Arrogance/Humility Paradigm." In that chapter, I discuss how important humility is in becoming wiser people and how arrogance can stand in the way of that process. The following is an excerpt from that chapter:

AUTHENTIC WISDOM VERSUS NAIVE WISDOM

AUTHENTIC WISDOM	NAIVE WISDOM
Many life experiences	Fewer life experiences
Based on humility	Can be arrogant
Loves to be a student	Has difficulty with continued learning
Understands reliance on the processes	Less reliance on the processes
Continues to move slowly	Has accelerated pace in life
Sees the bigger picture	Focus on smaller circumstances
Treats life as a journey	Sees some of the destination realized

DECEPTIVELY STRONG

Remember, the power you seek comes from others with more experience and expertise and from the program they represent and are trying to teach you. Humility keeps you connected with the program's power. It helps keep you from getting too full of yourself, which can happen with naive wisdom. As I define it, *Authentic wisdom cannot exist without humility.*

Arrogance and disconnecting from the people and programs that help you can interfere with your potential to learn and your ability to connect to others who can help facilitate the learning process that is so essential to recovery. It can become a true knowledge graveyard. Continued and sustained learning is crucial to recovery and, ultimately, to personal happiness and fulfillment.

Humility opens the door for continued personal growth and keeps you connected with power sources that fuel your journey. Arrogant people feel they have learned enough and do not need to continue to learn from others. Humble people understand that they can learn from others and that learning can improve their lives. Arrogance is the student who becomes the teacher and then refuses to continue being the student. Humility is the student who, while rising to the level of teacher, always remains a student of life.

It is so difficult for anyone with an arrogant disposition to let others in and take their advice. This is because it is so hard to trust other people with intimate information that may make us look weak and out of control and put us in a vulnerable position. Many people who struggle with letting others help them remain stuck in the addiction and in protecting the family secret, and they are destined to repeat this painful way of living each day.

BREAKING IT DOWN—THE ADDICT

It is easy to see how arrogance applies to the thoughts and behaviors of the addict. When an individual knowingly disregards the feelings of others, can be abusive, exhausts family resources, and generally displays little in the way of accountability for what they are doing, arrogance is easy to spot. Sometimes, the arrogance an addict displays is more subtle. They may do something wrong, quickly apologize, and maybe even mean what they say, but they quickly return to form and begin the behavioral pattern all over again.

For other addicts, arrogance is more readily observable. They can be angry, abusive, and, at times, violent. They will blame others for what the addiction has caused and almost seem to enjoy the make-believe power that they have over others. At times, they even seem to enjoy their little power trip and make it clear that they will not stop and no one can stop them. They accept no accountability and no responsibility to make any of the changes that are so necessary to save their lives and spare others the pain of their destruction.

Arrogance, however, can take on a more sinister presentation. Addicts can be subtle about their arrogance. Some of them are clever enough to realize that if they temper their arrogance with some quasi-sensitive behaviors, family members won't realize that they are being taken advantage of. The addict does gain the upper hand and keep family members and those close to them in their twisted service, but in the end, what they are doing is still arrogant, and their little diabolical scheme serves no purpose other than to keep them slaves to their own addiction.

BREAKING IT DOWN—FAMILY MEMBERS, LOVED ONES, AND SIGNIFICANT OTHERS

For family members and others close to the addict, it almost seems unfair to define them as arrogant. Referring back to the definition of "arrogance" from earlier in the chapter, arrogance is *an overbearing pride and haughtiness, demonstrating a perceived position of superiority.* Obviously, this directly defines the approach the addict uses. However, family members and friends are being victimized by the addiction. They are often left in a subordinate position, at times cowering to the addict's behaviors and attitude. How can they be seen as arrogant?

Family members may not seek help from others due to loyalties to the addict, fear of the addict, and fear of others' unjust judgments. As a result, they may refuse to allow others to help them. In the case of abuse and fear of retribution or harm from the addict, accepting help can be more difficult. However, loyalties to a person and life conditions that are dysfunctional and often abusive, or simply trying to protect the family's good name, are based on arrogance, though a much subtler form. Let's examine this a bit deeper.

Some family members feel that if they do all the right things, say all the right things, and be what they are supposed to be to the addict, the situation will eventually get better. This is where family members fool themselves into believing they have the power and the resources to fix the problem and the addict. This is rarely ever true, and since such family members have decided to fix this on their own, they do not seek the necessary help of people who know more than they do. In its truest form, this is a subtle form of arrogance, though it is not meant to hurt anyone. Since these family members and friends are trying to do this to help the addict, this has the semblance of altruistic caregiver behavior.

Consider this scenario: You are the friend of an addict and their family members. You know the family members are having a very difficult time. In your own life, you are recovering from the damage an addict has done to you. You have attended a counseling program and a 12-step group and have been in recovery for four or five years. You have experience regarding addiction, the knowledge you learned in counseling, and a support group and program always available to you. You reach out to help your friend. They tell you that you are wrong, the problem is not that bad, and they want to handle it independently. You already know that this will not happen. You try again and again, but your attempts are thwarted. You will probably leave the second conversation, saying they are making a grave mistake and that their pride and arrogance are keeping them from getting help. This, of course, assumes they are not in a position to be physically hurt by the addict.

Addiction, any way you cut it, is a very sick way to live life. People do desperate things in desperate times, and they can think and behave as though they are ill when they are caught up in circumstances surrounded by emotional, intellectual, and physical sickness. Unfortunately, for those caught up in the downward spiral that the addiction and the addict cause, there is a tendency to take on some of the addict's thoughts and behaviors and act accordingly. As with many other diseases, close contact is a contagious state of affairs. It is important to understand that life with an addict will change the way you think, feel, and behave. It's a case of not seeing the addictive forest because you are blinded by the addictive trees. It is vital to let other people in who can see the bigger picture.

MINIMUM IMPEDANCE EQUALS MAXIMUM GAINS

In Chapter 20, I discussed how recovery is an all-or-nothing proposition. There is no halfway with recovery. If you decide to dabble in recovery or do only some of the things that recovery demands, your potential for a successful recovery from the addiction will be seriously compromised. In the previous chapter, I made it clear that if you are serious about recovery from addiction, you must be willing to surrender to a program that can help you, to the people helping you, and to the advice they give you.

The greater the surrender and the less arrogance involved in the process, the more likely you are to leave the addiction behind. It is difficult to recover from the addiction and the addictive fallout all by yourself. Everyone needs help sometimes, and if you are in the throes of an addiction, whether you are the addict or someone close to them, you are part of that everyone. As you begin to work with a 12-step program, you enter the program not knowing much about recovery, follow the program to learn what to do, turn what you are learning into action, and finally turn your knowledge and experience into service to others. In the beginning stages of recovery, you do not know as much as you think you do about working through this problem. As you proceed in the program, surrender yourself to people who know more, learn about the program, and apply its principles. You will acquire the knowledge you need to maintain a healthy lifestyle.

Not surrendering, pride, arrogance, and any form of resistance impedes the efforts of the people helping you, and in the end, you can expect little change in the conditions of your life. However, as the title of this section suggests, minimum impedance—that is, with little resistance to the program as it is being explained to you—will garner the maximum results. The more you are willing to accept help from others on their terms, the closer you will come to that happy life you have been searching for.

So, here's the important question you need to ask yourself: "Do I need to feel as though I, myself, have all the information I need and can solve this problem on my own, or can I become a little more comfortable understanding that I do not have all the information or the plan to begin recovery, and I need the help of others to make this happen?" Those who can answer yes to needing more help are taking the first step in securing the people and the plan to begin a recovery program that can save their lives. You can do this. Be humble. Let others help.

 TIME TO TAKE ACTION

1. Refer to the chart that explains the difference between authentic and naive wisdom. See which applies more directly to you.

2. Be willing to put your pride and arrogance aside and begin asking other people questions about what is happening in your life. Be honest with them.

3. Assess your commitment to your recovery program. Be honest about this and be willing to examine it with the help of those who will assist you in moving forward in recovery.

4. Even if you do not understand or agree with the advice the experts give, be willing to discuss it with them, listen to what they have to say, and try to do what they suggest.

5. Understand the difference between real power and the mirage that addiction creates. Know that the only way to get the help you need is to let others help you. Present the facts to them, don't defend what you think you know, and start with a blank slate where you are willing to accept what the people who are trying to help you have to say to you. Make an honest attempt to incorporate their suggestions into your life.

DRIVING IT HOME

It can be difficult for anyone to leave something they are familiar with and then understand how to live without it. For the addict, there is the added difficulty of withdrawal from the addiction, the need to trust people you might perceive as out of touch, and following through on something others are suggesting when it's something you don't want to do. For family members, the challenge lies in understanding that you do not have the power to end the addict's addiction and that assuming you do only feeds into the addiction. Being humble enough to put your addiction-driven positions aside and start listening to those who know more and can help you is an important step in leaving the addiction behind and starting a new, productive, and happy life. Think about humility as the first step in power. If you take that step, the power you receive from others and the program that supports them can change your life.

YOUR DECLARATION IS: *I will be humbler and more willing to accept assistance from those who can help me!*

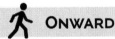 ## ONWARD

In the next chapter, I will discuss how to stay in today and keep your eyes firmly fixed on the prize, which in addiction recovery is sobriety. I will also discuss the mindset necessary to maintain this way of life.

CHAPTER 28

◇◇◇◇◇◇◇◇◇◇◇◇

Your New Life—No Setups; Eyes on the Prize

There are no cheats, shortcuts, or temporary escapes. Recovery is the powerful surrender and uncompromising commitment to your program, your higher power, yourself, your family, and everyone you touch.

PROCESSES TO EMPLOY: Brutal Honesty, I Over E, Present-Understand-Fix, Slowing Down Life's Pace, Internal Focus, Fact-Finding, Honesty, Patience, Truth-Telling, Belief, Listening, Trust, Reduction of Destination Living, Goal-Setting, Living in the Moment, One-Day-at-a-Time Living, Boundary-Setting, Warm Communication, Settling Past Issues, Risk-Taking, Be Comfortable with Being Uncomfortable, Humility, Gratitude, Faith, Dignity

---

THE OLD SAYING GOES THAT YOU GET OUT what you put in. In your recovery from the horrors of the addiction, this statement couldn't be more accurate. There is no easy way to walk away from the addiction and have everything be just right. Addictions typically take a reasonably long time to develop and reach their maximum level of damage. To assume that you could fix such a thing quickly or that recovery will be something you can learn fast would amount to nothing more than fooling yourself. Entering recovery and learning how to stay there will take time, and it will take effort. The more you put into it, the better the results.

Let's summarize what you must do to start your recovery plan. In Chapter 19, I began providing the information you will need to start building your recovery program. If you are going to be successful in setting up your plan, you know you will need to:

1. Decide that you are going to separate yourself from the addiction and begin a recovery program.

2. Make an appointment with your primary care physician to determine if there are any physical concerns.

3. Make an appointment with an addiction specialist to gather information about your circumstances.

4. Look into a 12-step program and contact someone there to begin the support component for your program.

A good recovery program begins with these four steps. Refer to the information I provided in Chapters 19 through 27 for the expanded details of how to get your program started. It is understandable to want to separate yourself from the addiction and begin your happy life as quickly as possible. Nothing about the addiction is enjoyable, and no one would fault you for wanting to live a happy, healthy life as soon as you can. However, there can be serious consequences when you try too fast. Recovery from an addiction is a step-by-step process for both the addict and their family members, loved ones, and significant others. There are no shortcuts; skipping steps can become nothing more than setups for relapses.

Try to look at each step in their recovery process as a learning process. Each step teaches you something about the addiction, what you were thinking and feeling, how you behaved during that time, and some practical measures to help you address those specific issues. Each step is also a bridge to the next step. This means that each step you learn introduces you to the next step while helping you cross over with enough knowledge and resources to begin to address the work that needs to be done in the new step. This is why the step-by-step, day-to-day approach is so important.

If you are willing to surrender to knowledgeable people and a workable program, you will be guided through each step, which will help you connect your current step with the one that follows it. Your supporters will help you when you get stuck or have difficulty, and your program guides will keep you from going too fast. Working with them and acquiescing to their expertise keeps you grounded in the program, and as this happens, you will begin to trust them and your daily step-by-step recovery program.

THE CHEATS AND THE SHORTCUTS

For some people, patience is anything but a virtue; they tend to attach timetables and deadlines to their recovery program, and they, themselves, determine when they have reached these destinations. These destinations usually have more to do with immediate gratification, feeling good, and working less than they do with understanding the information each step of the program provides and working those steps to one's maximum recovery potential. Immediate gratification is one of the dysfunctional attributes that makes addiction work. You see it, you want it, and you do whatever is necessary to acquire it as soon as possible.

Of course, this does not lead to sustained recovery. It does not allow for appropriate time to understand the information you need to address the addiction and learn how to live in recovery. It also doesn't provide enough time for that sustained connection to your program guide, counselor, or sponsor, which is essential to keeping you moving forward in the program. Let's look at some cheats and shortcuts people use, sometimes consciously and sometimes without understanding they are using them:

➤ Reapplying the advice to fit your needs without consulting your guide to ensure it is the right decision.

➤ Taking some of your guide's advice, but not all of it.

➤ For addicts, merely reducing your involvement with your drug or activity of choice but telling everyone else that you have completely stopped.

➤ For family members, telling those who are advising you that you are not enabling the addict when you are still doing things to keep them happy.

➤ Telling others you are doing all the work when you know you are only doing part of it.

➤ Deciding that it is acceptable to use (the addict) or enable (family members) once in a while so you can feel relief from the accountability the program demands.

➤ For addicts, using a different drug or activity as a substitute for the drug or activity of choice. For example, instead of snorting methamphetamine, the addict might use considerably more caffeine, energy drinks, and other amphetamine-based substances to get their high, or they might refrain from trips to the casino only to increase their purchases of lottery tickets.

➤ For family members, substituting new enabling behaviors to help convince themselves that they are no longer supporting the addict's game plan. For example, they may stop trying to convince the addict to refrain from using their drug or activity of choice and instead either be overly receptive to their needs or use passive-aggressive methods to get their point across.

➤ The most damaging cheat is telling your guide you're doing what they are suggesting when you're not turning their advice into action.

You may note that your involvement with your program guide is missing in these examples, so you would be making these decisions on your own and without their knowledge. Isn't this what you did before you involved yourself in your recovery program? Isn't keeping secrets, not taking anyone else's advice, and making your own decisions to keep you happy in the moment what got you into this mess? In all these examples, and any others that do not include your program guide's involvement, these decisions are typically made because you know your guides will advise you not to do what you are planning to do.

This is where defense mechanisms often come into play. "Defense mechanisms" are *unconscious strategies that help people protect themselves from anxious thoughts or feelings, from admitting the truth, and from being accountable for one's actions.* There are many, but let's look at those that lend themselves to program cheats and shortcuts.

- **DENIAL**—This is where you deny or are unwilling to admit that you are doing what you are being confronted with. In denial, the addict or family member is not taking ownership of what they are doing to support the addiction, even though their actions demonstrate the opposite to those who are trying to help them.

- **INTELLECTUALIZATION**—This is where addicts and family members provide what they believe is an intelligent reason to continue doing things in a way that supports the addiction. They might try to convince you that there are benefits to doing things the way they are doing them. The compulsive gambler may try to convince you that the big score will significantly enhance the lives of the family members. In contrast, family members might say that the money the addicts are spending comes from sources that render it "disposable income" and that other family needs are still being met.

- **RATIONALIZATION**—This is the practice of using excuses and alternative reasons to cover up facts and motives. The addict may say that if they stop the addiction completely, something terrible is going to happen. Family members may talk about painful repercussions if they stop performing their supportive behaviors.

- **REPRESSION**—Unconsciously keeping unpleasant information from your conscious mind. This is where both the addict and family members compartmentalize or do their best not to think about what is happening.

ALL OR NOTHING—NO CHEATS AND NO SHORTCUTS

In Chapter 20, I discussed how addiction residue is the intellectual and sometimes physical craving that pulls you back into the active phase of the addiction. If the commitment to recovery isn't all or nothing, it leaves the brain and the body caught between the halfhearted attempt at recovery and the obsessive chase for euphoria attached to the addiction. In the early stages of recovery, this is precisely what's happening. You may be desperately trying to move forward, leave the addiction behind, and begin a new way to live your life, but the addiction keeps pulling at you, and at times, its draw may be difficult to ignore.

Without realizing it, you begin to keep secrets and avoid your program guides. You find reasons to avoid sessions and meetings, stop contacting them, find reasons why the program is either too difficult or not working for you, or argue that the program guide doesn't understand you. Remember, you cannot serve two masters. If you are going to navigate through this unknown recovery territory successfully, it will be with the help of those who know more and know how to help you. Your first red flag is your reduced involvement with your counselor, sponsor, and other support people. There are always ways to stay in touch with them. Let them know what is happening in your life and let them help you. Always keep yourself close to your program guides. They are your most important lifeline to your recovery plan, and staying close to them is critical.

THE FOUR STEPS OF ALL-IN PROGRAM INVOLVEMENT

1. Promise yourself that nothing will interfere with your continued involvement with your program guide and your program.

2. Attend all counseling sessions and support meetings without reservation and with 100% commitment to do what you are advised. Make no excuses.

3. Do not keep secrets from your program guides. Tell them everything that is happening in your life according to the schedule they set for you.

4. Understand that your recovery program is a plan you will use for the rest of your life. Your level of involvement will be determined in conjunction with your program guide, but working in an intelligent program means staying involved in that program and using its steps and traditions to guide you into that happy life you were looking for and to help you stay there.

"All or nothing" seems like a demanding way to live life, an unyielding taskmaster. It is a life of accountability, commitment, trust, and honesty. There is work to be done, but many people are willing to help you along the way. Too many of us shy away from commitment and accountability because we feel it keeps us boxed in and constrained, prisoners in an onerous way to live. Recovery is anything but. Addiction robs everyone involved of the clear, disciplined thought that paves the way for a happy life. Intelligent life decisions are based on sound information and thoughtfully executed planning. A recovery program is nothing but a disciplined program that gives you the information you need to help you point your life in the direction that leads to happiness.

A recovery program always has counselors, sponsors, and guides willing to ease you into this disciplined way of living, to help you remove what doesn't work, and to be there for you through the entire process. This is a new-life family. The love is unconditional, and the commitment is without question. However, there is one simple catch: You must be all in. On a hot, oppressive day, you can't feel the relief from the cool waters of a swimming pool until you get all in. In life, you cannot feel the relief from the oppression that comes from the addiction until you completely immerse yourself in your recovery program and stay close to those who are guiding you. If you do, a wonderful new life is waiting for you. Be committed, be willing to do the work, open up to others, and don't back down. Get all in, and stay all in. Your program guides are waiting to wrap their arms around you. You can do this!

 TIME TO TAKE ACTION

1. Commit to be all in your recovery program.

2. Attend all counseling sessions and support meetings.

3. Be completely honest with your program guides.

4. Establish a contact protocol with your program guides and contact them as often as possible.

5. Make the "Four Steps of All-In Program Involvement" your personal commitment to yourself in your recovery program.

6. If you are having difficulty with your program, have slipped back and returned to some old bad habits, or have been away for a while, call your program guide and get back into the program flow. There are no judgments in recovery, only love and respect. You will be welcomed back.

 ## DRIVING IT HOME

When you were in the grasp of the addiction, you were in the grasp of a painful and prison-like existence. Entering your recovery program can change your life and rescue you from the horrors of the addiction, and it requires an all-in attitude. If you are willing to make the commitment the program requires, a much happier life is waiting for you. There is work to be done, and nothing worth having comes without work. This step-by-step, day-by-day program for life will help you break the addiction chains that have so drastically affected your life. *Be all in to your recovery. Be all in to the program. Be all in to your program guides.* If you do, you will allow them to be all in for you, and this is when life gets good.

YOUR DECLARATION IS: *I will invest myself in my recovery program, stay close to those who are guiding me, and do what they tell me to do to live a sober and healthy life!*

 ## ONWARD

In the next chapter, as in all the final chapters in The Fix Yourself Empowerment Series, I will discuss housekeeping as it applies to keeping yourself honest and committed to sobriety. I will also discuss slips, return visitors, and, when you have been absent from those who can help you, your necessary return to the program that can save your life.

CHAPTER 29

Good Housekeeping— Recovery's Best Friend

It is sobriety's checks and balances. It says, "I will never be done." It is the never-ending recovery gift that keeps on giving.

PROCESSES TO EMPLOY: Brutal Honesty, I Over E, Present-Understand-Fix, Slowing Down Life's Pace, Internal Focus, Fact-Finding, Honesty, Patience, Truth-Telling, Belief, Listening, Trust, Reduction of Destination Living, Goal-Setting, Living in the Moment, One-Day-at-a-Time Living, Boundary-Setting, Warm Communication, Settling Past Issues, Risk-Taking, Be Comfortable with Being Uncomfortable, Humility, Gratitude, Faith, Dignity, Housekeeping

---

WHEN IT COMES TO THE WORK we all need to do in our lives, we like to get to a point where we know we are done, when we have reached our work destination, when we can sit back and relax and reflect on a job well done. We would like to know that a job will take a particular amount of time and effort, that there is a goal in mind, and that when we achieve that goal, we can be done with the work. We want to finish the job and never need to go back and start again. We don't want to hear that there is no destination, that the work will be a lifetime affair, and that there is no finish line.

Unfortunately, recovery from addiction doesn't work that way. Addiction always seems to be waiting just around the corner in case we make a mistake and unlock that recovery door. If we do decide to let our guard down and take a break from our program, we can expect some of those old thoughts and behaviors to return, and the problems could range from a simple backward regression to the return to a full-blown addiction and everything that goes with it.

In every book I have written and every program I have presented as I counsel people, and in The Fix Yourself Empowerment Series, I stress the notion of housekeeping. Think of it in terms of the way you maintain your home. If you throw a big party and the house gets trashed, a few things are broken, the floors are sticky, dishes and glasses are everywhere, and the whole place smells like the inside of an outhouse on a hot day, you want to clean that mess up as fast as you can, and you never want it to return to that state again.

To keep your home clean and problem-free, it is important to do routine maintenance. This keeps things in order and your home life comfortable and, for the most part, problem-free. Your addiction housekeeping program is similar in its design. You are doing what you must to keep yourself in a program of recovery that helps ensure your health and happiness. To make this program work, it is important to give it continued attention. If you do, you reduce the threat of the addiction returning and your life falling, once again, into disarray.

I have been stressing that your recovery will be a lifetime program for you. This doesn't mean that you will be hard at work every day of your life. There is much work to be done at the beginning of your recovery. Still, as you progress to the point that the addiction is no longer active and you have secured all the necessary program guides who can be there for you for the rest of your life, it is simply a matter of continuing to work on the steps of your program to the best of your ability.

You may continue to attend meetings and occasionally return for counseling sessions for a bit of a tune-up. At other times, the addiction may rear its ugly head to some degree, either on your part or on the part of someone close to you. In that case, it may be time to bear down, go back to basics, and reinvolve yourself with the program more intensely. When you think about it, it's far more appealing to continue to maintain your status in the program than it is to return to the pain the addiction causes in its active stages.

In the clutches of the addiction, life runs on autopilot. I discussed this concept in detail in *The Fix Yourself Handbook*. Running on autopilot means you stop applying enough conscious energy to what you are doing and make thoroughly considered decisions in favor of disengaging your brain, like a pilot using the plane's autopilot feature to fly. The plane keeps flying, but the pilot is not actively controlling its movement. This is what happens in the case of addiction-instigated autopilot living. The addiction runs the show, and you follow along without enough thought or a plan to make changes when necessary.

Your housekeeping efforts are nothing more than returning to conscious thought and looking at the information honestly and efficiently. This allows you to get help when necessary and make sound decisions that can positively impact your life as you are living it today and for the rest of your life. It is a program that is invaluable, whether you are recovering from addiction or simply living your day-to-day life. Conscious thought and daily maintenance keep you grounded and aware of what is happening around you and when you need help.

Try not to think of housekeeping as a lifetime chore that will remove you from all the fun life offers. This couldn't be farther from the truth. Housekeeping keeps you involved with your program guides. Continue to go to meetings. Stay close to the people who initially helped you through the difficult times. Never become arrogant enough to believe you have "arrived" and do not need the program anymore. The program and your guides are what changed your life. Stay humble and stay close to them. Look at housekeeping and your continued involvement in your recovery program and with the people who helped you as a marvelous gift, one that can keep you grounded, connected, and happy for the rest of your life.

Your life is a dynamic process. It will change year to year and, in some cases, day to day. There is no guarantee that all the gains you are making will remain constant and that addiction, or some part of it, won't rear its ugly head from time to time. The addiction was horrible, and you took the steps to open your life to a program and to the people involved in it who showed you a new way to live and helped you change your life. Return visits are fixable if you stay close to your program and those helping you. Whether it is maintaining a healthy life on a routine basis by staying close to the program or fixing a slip or relapse, the program will always be there for you, and you will always be able to clean your recovery house. You did it once, and you'll do it again. It is reassuring to know that regardless of what happens, there is a program "safety net" under you with people ensuring it is secure enough to hold the weight of your pain. Take comfort in that.

THE NEVER-ENDING STORY

Housekeeping is an ongoing state of affairs, a process of checks and balances that never stops. All happy people must adjust, transition, and defend their gains routinely. Know that if you remain committed to the program and the processes I have been teaching you to use, the external world becomes that much less oppressive. Housekeeping is one of those processes. When you use it, all return visitors are assigned to the new, stronger version of you, and the negative and toxic invaders will perish there. Follow these steps and keep your program life house strong.

THE 7 STEPS FOR SUCCESSFUL HOUSECLEANING

1. Be ready for return visitors; they are coming.

2. Identify your new intruder.

3. Include your program guides and be honest about what you are reporting.

4. Slow down and keep your emotions in check.

5. Gather all the necessary facts.

6. Based on the facts, let your program supports help you to develop a plan to address the problem. Use your counselor, program guides, or sponsors and the information I have been teaching in this book to address the problem.

7. Execute your plan completely; use your program and your support people.

You made the bravest decision of your life when you decided to let someone in to help you work through the addiction that was terrorizing your life and the lives of those close to you. Then you did all the work to settle old issues and learn how to think, feel, and behave without all the addiction insanity. Embracing the need for help, getting the help, and doing what you needed to do to remove the pain from your life was the hard part. Know that housekeeping and keeping your guides close to you can save your life. Treat this as the wonderful gift it is. Staying in touch with your guides and working with your program daily is not a chore—It is indeed a gift that keeps on giving.

Previously, you had no program or support system to help you. You do now. In the past, you were alone, defeated, and without options. You are no longer alone; you have become stronger, and you have options. Treat the addiction's returned visit, or any negative energy, as something you took care of previously and which you can take care of again. The need for housekeeping never indicates that you have moved backward, failed, or are doing things incorrectly. Housekeeping is a wonderful reminder that you have the strength to once again remove the addiction from your world and continue living the loving, peaceful life you are creating.

 TIME TO TAKE ACTION

1. Understand that your program is a program for life and that staying close to your program guides and counselors is essential. Stay in contact with them.

2. Your program steps are valuable methods for helping you recover from addiction. They are also your guide to a happy, healthy life. Use them every day.

3. Each evening, consciously review what occurred during your day. Ask yourself if any parts of the addiction or the life you previously led in the active grasp of the addiction influenced the course of your life that day.

4. Discuss any changes in your life with your program guides and supports, regardless of how small those changes are. It's not only about opening your life in the early stages of recovery. It's about always keeping your life open.

5. Never feel as though you have arrived at your recovery destination. Live every day with a healthy recovery plan that addresses everyone and everything that enters your life during that day.

 DRIVING IT HOME

While you may be tempted to view housekeeping as another chore you must perform to keep the addiction from reentering your world, try not to think of it that way. Housekeeping is a wonderful process tool that is always available to keep you from reverting to old habits and experiencing the pain that can come from doing so. Use it to address the issues from the addiction and for everything else in your life. Become someone who routinely evaluates what you are doing and how to do it better. Housekeeping reminds you how strong you are. It can be used not only to keep the addiction from reentering your world but also as checks and balances that can be applied to every part of your life. Treat it as the gift it is, and keep your world positive, loving, and productive. Remember, you are a beautiful person. Be that person!

YOUR DECLARATION IS: *I will do my housekeeping every day of my life. I will keep my program and program guides close, and I will be happy!*

ONWARD!

Conclusion

THERE ARE MANY DIFFERENT TYPES OF ADDICTION. All of them can have damaging effects ranging from mild to devastating. Unless you live on a deserted island, all addictions can result in collateral damage. Nothing about addiction is easy. It can lock you in a world of pain and secrecy. It can rob you of your dignity, family and friends, resources, and health. It can lay waste to the minds and hearts of the best of us and tear healthy, loving families to shreds.

There is hope for those willing to share what is happening in their lives and open themselves up to caring people eager to help them. Recovery will not be easy. If it were easy, everyone would be doing it. However, *nothing* about recovery is impossible. The most important point to remember is that your willingness to accept help from people who are more experienced with addiction recovery and who have the resources and expertise to help you is invaluable in your recovery.

Be willing to let in the people who know how to help you, listen to what they are saying, take their advice, and work with the step-by-step plan they provide. Remember, nothing about recovery is halfway. It's an all-or-nothing proposition. Get all in, and stay all in. When times get tough, your support people and your program will be there for you.

Recovery is a lifetime program, and it is a program that will be there for you for your entire life. The addiction made you feel alone, without direction and hope. The program and the people in it will provide direction; they will always be there for you, and you will have hope. Make the call. Let them in. Listen to them. Take their advice, and learn to be happy. You are beautiful, and you deserve all the good things in life. YOU CAN DO THIS!

Endnotes

(1) Ruggiero, Faust, M.S. *The Fix Yourself Handbook*. Bangor, Pa. FYHB Publications. 2023

(2) Ruggiero, Faust, M.S. *The Fix Your Anxiety Handbook*. Bangor, Pa. FYHB Publications. 2023

(3) Ruggiero, Faust, M.S. *The Fix Your Depression Handbook*. Bangor, Pa. FYHB Publications. 2023

(4) Ruggiero, Faust, M.S. *The Fix Your Anger Handbook*. Bangor, Pa. FYHB Publications. 2024

(5) National Institute on Alcohol Abuse and Alcoholism, Alcohol Facts and Statistics: https://www.niaaa.nih.gov/sites/default/files/publications/NIAAA_Alcohol_Facts_and_Stats_0.pdf, 2019

(6) National Institute on Drug Abuse, Tobacco, Nicotine, and E-Cigarettes Research Report: https://nida.nih.gov/publications/research-reports/tobacco-nicotine-e-cigarettes/what-scope-tobacco-use-its-cost-to-society#:~:-text=22.0%25%20(or%20about%2061.6%20million,days%20(2021%20DT%202.1), 2021

(7) National Centers for Drug Abuse Statistics, Drug Abuse Statistics: https://drugabusestatistics.org/, 2020

(8) Centers for Disease Control, Heroin: https://www.cdc.gov/overdose-prevention/ about/heroin.html, 2022

(9) Addiction Help.com, Cocaine Addiction Statistics: https://www.addictionhelp.com/cocaine/statistics/

(10) National Institute on Drug Abuse, What is the scope of methamphetamine use in the United States?: https://nida.nih.gov/publications/

research-reports/methamphetamine/what-scope-methamphetamine-misuse-in-united-states, 2019

(11) Newport Institute, Hallucinogen Use in Young Adults: New Stats and Research: https://www.newportinstitute.com/resources/co-occurring-disorders/young-adult-hallucinogen-use/, 2023

(12) Centers for Disease Control, Cannabis Facts and Stats: https://www.cdc.gov/cannabis/data-research/facts-stats/index.html, 2021

(13) Addiction Help.com, The Changing Landscape of Food Addiction: https://www.addictionhelp.com/food-addiction/statistics/, 2024

(14) Quit Gambling.com, Gambling Addiction Statistics & Facts 2024: https://quitgamble.com/gambling-addiction-statistics-and-facts/#ib-toc-anchor-0, 2024

(15) Reviews.org, Cell Phone Usage Statistics: Mornings Are for Notifications: https://www.reviews.org/mobile/cell-phone-addiction/, 2023

(16) Game Quitters.com, Video Game Addiction Statistics 2023—How Many Addicted Gamers Are There?: https://gamequitters.com/video-game-addiction-statistics/, 2023

(17) Bed Bible.com, Sexual Addiction Statistics: 24 Eye-Opening Facts: https://bedbible.com/sex-addiction-statistics/, 2024

(18) Centers for Disease Control, Suicide and Self-Harm Injury: https://www.cdc.gov/nchs/fastats/suicide.htm, 2024

(19) Addiction Help.com, Shopping Addiction Statistics- https://www.addictionhelp.com/shopping-addiction/statistics/, 2024

(20) Very Well Mind, Shopping Addiction Statistics: https://www.verywellmind.com/shopping-addiction-4157288, 2023

(21) Clockify, Workaholism facts and statistics: everything you need to know: https://clockify.me/workaholism-facts, 2024

(22) Addiction Help.com, Helping You From Addiction to Recovery: https://www.addictionhelp.com/, 2024

(23) Pub Med; The Harvard Twin Study: h*ttps://pubmed.ncbi.nlm.nih.gov/11600486/, 2021*

References

1 Pub Med; The Harvard Twin Study: https://pubmed.ncbi.nlm.nih.gov/11600486/, 2021

2 National Institute on Alcohol Abuse and Alcoholism, Alcohol Facts and Statistics: https://www.niaaa.nih.gov/sites/default/files/publications/NIAAA_Alcohol_Facts_and_Stats_0.pdf, 2019

3 National Institute on Alcohol Abuse and Alcoholism, Alcohol Facts and Statistics: https://www.niaaa.nih.gov/sites/default/files/publications/NIAAA_Alcohol_Facts_and_Stats_0.pdf, 2019

4 National Centers for Drug Abuse Statistics, Drug Abuse Statistics: https://drugabusestatistics.org/, 2020

5 Centers for Disease Control, Heroin: https://www.cdc.gov/overdose-prevention/about/heroin.html, 2022

6 Addiction Help.com, Cocaine Addiction Statistics: https://www.addictionhelp.com/cocaine/statistics/

7 National Institute on Drug Abuse, What is the scope of methamphetamine use in the United States?: https://nida.nih.gov/publications/research-reports/methamphetamine/what-scope-methamphetamine-misuse-in-united-states, 2019

8 Newport Institute, Hallucinogen Use in Young Adults: New Stats and Research: https://www.newportinstitute.com/resources/co-occurring-disorders/young-adult-hallucinogen-use/, 2023

9 Centers for Disease Control, Cannabis Facts and Stats: https://www.cdc.gov/cannabis/data-research/facts-stats/index.html, 2021

10 Addiction Help.com, The Changing Landscape of Food Addiction: https://www.addictionhelp.com/food-addiction/statistics/, 2024

11 Addiction Help.com, The Changing Landscape of Food Addiction: https://www.addictionhelp.com/food-addiction/statistics/, 2024

12 Quit Gambling.com, Gambling Addiction Statistics & Facts 2024: https://quitgamble.com/gambling-addiction-statistics-and-facts/#ib-toc -anchor-0, 2024

13 Reviews.org, Cell Phone Usage Statistics: Mornings Are for Notifications: https://www.reviews.org/mobile/cell-phone-addiction/, 2023

14 Game Quitters.com, Video Game Addiction Statistics 2023—How Many Addicted Gamers Are There?: https://gamequitters.com/video-game -addiction-statistics/, 2023

15 Bed Bible.com, Sexual Addiction Statistics: 24 Eye-Opening Facts: https://bedbible.com/sex-addiction-statistics/, 2024

16 Centers for Disease Control, Suicide and Self-Harm Injury: https:// www.cdc.gov/nchs/fastats/suicide.htm, 2024

17 Addiction Help.com, Shopping Addiction Statistics https://www .addictionhelp.com/shopping-addiction/statistics/, 2024

18 Clockify, Workaholism facts and statistics: everything you need to know: https://clockify.me/workaholism-facts, 2024

19 https://www.healthline.com/health/exercise-addiction#symptoms

20 Addiction Help.com, Helping You From Addiction to Recovery: https:// www.addictionhelp.com/, 2024

About the Author

FAUST A. RUGGIERO'S professional career spans over forty years of diversified, cutting-edge counseling programs pursuing professional excellence and personal life enhancement. He is a published research author, clinical trainer, and therapist with experience in clinics for deaf children, prisons, nursing homes, substance abuse centers, inpatient facilities, and major national and international corporations. He has served as the president of the Community Psychological Center in Bangor, Pennsylvania. In that capacity, he developed the Process Way of Life counseling program, later presented as a formal text in *The Fix Yourself Handbook*.

Upon graduating from Mansfield University in 1977, he enrolled in the graduate psychology program at Illinois State University with a dual major in clinical and developmental psychology and a minor in research. He assisted in the publication of several research articles, including his thesis, "The Effects of Prosocial and Antisocial Television Programs on the Cognitions of Children."

Upon leaving graduate school in 1979, Mr. Ruggiero worked with Antoinette Goffredo to provide counseling services and psychological intervention to adolescent deaf children and to develop a behavioral management program for profoundly deaf children with residual hearing.

In 1982, he accepted a position with the Lehigh Valley Alcohol Counseling Center. There, he provided individual counseling services to clientele suffering from alcohol abuse and addiction, including the 12-step recovery process and family and intervention services. There, Mr. Ruggiero developed a Phase 2 counseling program for individuals convicted of drunk-driving offenses.

In 1984, he accepted a treatment position at Northampton County Prison, where he provided psychological and substance abuse intake and counseling services. He coordinated all substance abuse and program development services for inmates. In 1986, he obtained his certification in substance abuse treatment in the state of Pennsylvania.

In 1989, Mr. Ruggiero left Northampton County prison to pursue his endeavors at the Community Psychological Center full-time. As president of the Community Psychological Center, Mr. Ruggiero continued to provide services to individuals, families, those suffering from substance abuse, abused women, and women in transition, as well as couples and marriage counseling and counseling for veterans, law enforcement, and other first responders. In 1990, he began providing employee assistance programs to corporations in the state of Pennsylvania. Since then, he has been nationally and internationally recognized for his business approaches to strengthening corporate administrators and their workforces. In 1994, Mr. Ruggiero accepted an invitation to become a trainer for the Department of Health in Pennsylvania.

Following several years of experimentation with various therapeutic approaches that could be applied to clients individually and in families, social relationships, and business and corporate settings, Mr. Ruggiero developed and employed the Process Way of Life Counseling Program. The program consists of over fifty internal human processes, which can be accessed and developed to help clients address the various conditions affecting their lives. The program was developed, rigorously researched and tested, and revised into the approach he presently uses at the Community Psychological Center.

In the summer of 2016, Mr. Ruggiero began to develop *The Fix Yourself Empowerment Series* based on the Process Way of Life Program to help readers address the difficult situations in their lives. The award-winning *The Fix Yourself Handbook* was completed in December 2019. He has appeared on television, radio shows, and podcasts, both national and international, to discuss the Process Way of Life. His radio show—*Fix It With Faust,* debuted in June 2021. On June 8, 2023, the second installment in The Fix Yourself Empowerment Series, *The Fix Your Anxiety Handbook*, was published. It is also an award-winning publication. In December 2023, *The Fix Your Depression Handbook*, the third book in the series, was published. The *Fix Your Anger Handbook*, the series' fourth book, was published in May 2024.

Made in the USA
Middletown, DE
27 May 2025

76160680R00186